Integral Recovery

SUNY Series in Integral Theory

Sean Esbjörn-Hargens, editor

Integral Recovery

A Revolutionary Approach to the
Treatment of Alcoholism and Addiction

JOHN DUPUY

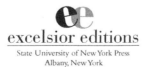

excelsior editions

State University of New York Press
Albany, New York

Cover photo of "Tall Aspens" courtesy of Zach Hessler / www.naturesgiftphotography.com

Published by State University of New York Press, Albany

Excelsior Editions is an imprint of State University of New York Press

For information, contact State University of New York Press, Albany, NY
www.sunypress.edu

Production by Ryan Morris
Marketing by Kate McDonnell

Library of Congress Cataloging-in-Publication Data

Dupuy, John, 1956–
    Integral recovery : a revolutionary approach to the treatment of alcoholism and addiction / John Dupuy.
        p. cm. — (Excelsior editions)
    Includes bibliographical references and index.
    ISBN 978-1-4384-4613-4 (hardcover : alk. paper)
    ISBN 978-1-4384-4614-1 (pbk. : alk. paper)
    1. Alcoholism—Treatment.   2. Substance abuse—Treatment.   3. Psychotherapy.
I. Title.

    RC565.D87 2013
    616.86'0651—dc23   2012017396

Contents

Illustrations

that addiction *is* a brain disease. Also, thanks to Bill Harris and Holosync® for being such a big part of my initial healing journey.

I am also grateful to my dear and beloved partner in iAwake Technologies, Eric Thompson, for your genius, huge heart, and friendship. You are a game-changer, and I love you. Thank you also to Jane Bunker, for saying yes to this book. Finally, thank you to all my students and their families. You have been my greatest teachers.

And, last but not least, thank you, God, I'm really grateful.

Illustrations

Acknowledgments

It is a pleasure to be able to publicly thank and honor those who made me possible, and those who made the writing of this book possible. First, I would like to acknowledge my parents. When I was in graduate school, we did three quarters of group therapy, and during that process I claimed that I had really good parents and that all my personal problems were my own. My fellow students all thought I was in denial, but that's my story and I'm sticking to it. I love you, Mom and Dad.

I want to give thanks to my wife, Pam, who gave me the time and space to write this book—see, I told you! And thank you to Heidi Mitchell, my assistant, who fell in love with this project early on and became my constant confidante, editor, support person, and mirror. Toward the end of the writing of this book, I would pace the floor and dictate to Heidi, and the atmosphere of trust, humor, and intelligence that was generated in our working together is something I will always be grateful for. And I want to do it again, Heidi.

Thank you to all my family members; my brothers, Rick and Frank; my children, John and Tina; and my beloved nephews, Romeo and Adrian. You have all been life shapers. Thank you, Adrian, for your courage, and thank you Romeo for all the tears and laughter.

I give thanks to all my Integral friends and teachers, starting, of course, with Ken Wilber for punching a big fat whole in the universe that the rest of us could follow you through. To Marco Morelli, thank you for helping to organize my thoughts early on. You are the kick in the pants that I needed. Thank you to Dennis Wittrock, Leslie Hershberger, David Riordan, Jennifer Walton, Diane Hamilton, Shawn Phillips, Dr. Adam Gorman, and Brother David Stendl-Rast (for healing my broken Christian heart; the hug did go back forty years). And thank you to Dr. Kevin McCauley for your pioneering work in helping us to understand that addiction *is* a brain disease. Also, thanks to Bill Harris and Holosync® for being such a big part of my initial healing journey.

I am also grateful to my dear and beloved partner in iAwake Technologies, Eric Thompson, for your genius, huge heart, and friendship. You are a game-changer, and I love you. Thank you also to Jane Bunker, for saying yes to this book. Finally, thank you to all my students and their families. You have been my greatest teachers.

And, last but not least, thank you, God, I'm really grateful.

Introduction

Why Another Book on Recovery from Addiction?

Chances are if you are reading this, there's an addict in your life. Maybe it's a family member, a friend, a client, a co-worker. Maybe it's you. For years, I have worked on the front lines of addiction treatment, working with families and individuals. This journey has taken me to the inside of jails, hospitals, AA meetings, wilderness quests, juvenile halls, funeral parlors, and countless other environments, where the toll of the disease can be seen in the naked suffering that it causes. In the case of my brother, addiction to pharmaceuticals coupled with depression led to his suicide; a beloved aunt died a slow, painful death of emphysema from a lifetime of smoking; and an uncle who had struggled with alcoholism for years ended his life with a shotgun. This is just a small part of *my* story. Each of you reading this will have your own stories and losses.

I hope it will be evident in the course of this book that the circle of our concern and care is not just for the suffering addict, but for all who have suffered from the ravages of this disease. When you begin to look comprehensively at addiction and make the connections to neglected and abused children, fetal alcohol syndrome, crimes committed, individuals locked up, suicides, families destroyed, talents and gifts never realized, and hopes dashed, the extent of the suffering you find is simply enormous. It is my hope and prayer that this book and Integral Recovery can begin to shine a new light of hope where before there has existed largely confusion and despair. This book is intended to work on the front lines of the fight against the disease of addiction: in the hands of addicts and their families, their loved ones, their health care providers, their therapists, their friends, their teachers and life coaches. Integral Recovery is about action, about practice, about commitment, and about service—not merely an intellectual exercise or discourse on a philosophical approach

1

(although it can be that too)—but something for you to study and then engage in, to move upon the knowledge. Integral Recovery is an urgent appeal to stand up, reach out, and set foot on the journey of recovery, self-discovery, and transformation.

As Americans, we must begin by asking the question, Why do we (the United States) use the lion's share of the illegal drugs on the planet, when we are such a small percentage of the population? What is going on, and what went wrong? Why has our war on drugs, which started as far back as the Nixon administration, failed to stop the spread and rise of drug use and abuse in our country, among all age groups and socioeconomic groups? Another way of putting this is, Why haven't we been able to protect generations of our children from drugs, tobacco, and alcohol?

Some years ago, I was trying to connect these dots on a personal level as well as at the larger national and world levels. At one point, I thought this might be a book I had to write. Happily, someone beat me to the punch. *High Society*,[1] a recently published book by Joseph A. Califano Jr., former director of the Department of Health, Education, and Welfare under Jimmy Carter, brilliantly illuminates the price that our civilization, culture, economy, families, and individuals are paying for the plague of drug abuse and addiction that is wreaking havoc on our country and our world. Califano does a masterful job of laying out the costs and causes of this human catastrophe in a clarion call of alarm and possible hope—if we change our attitudes and approaches to the myriad issues involving drug abuse and addiction in our country. "Although we are 4% of the world's population, we Americans consume 65 percent of the world's illegal drugs. One in four Americans will have an alcohol or drug disorder at some point in his or her life. And most of these people have parents, children, siblings, friends, and colleagues who will suffer collateral damage."[2]

Califano's call is to sober up our "High Society" and to recognize that substance abuse and addiction together make up "the nation's number one serial killer and crippler." And he calls for us to acknowledge these fundamental realities:

- Addiction is a chronic disease of epidemic proportions, with physical, psychological, emotional, and spiritual elements that require continuing and holistic [Integral] care.

- Addiction is a culprit implicated in our nation's high health care costs, crime, and social ills, including child abuse and neglect, chronic poverty, homelessness, teen pregnancy, the wildfire spread of sexually transmitted diseases, and family breakup.

• There are statistical and biological (chemical and neuro-logical) relationships among smoking, abusing alcohol, and marijuana use, and between abuse of those drugs and use of cocaine, heroin, prescription drugs, methamphetamines, hallucinogens, and other substances.

According to the National Institute on Drug Abuse, the economic cost of drug abuse in the United States reaches into the hundreds of billions of dollars.[3] In 2006, the Schneider Institute[4] estimated that 10 percent of the National Health Care Budget was being spent on drug abuse and addiction: $230 billion and climbing every year. Hold this thought in the light and add to it that only around 10 percent of those who need treatment actually get it and that even in the blue chip treatment centers the success rates are approximately 30 percent.[5] We can begin to see the magnitude of the problem. Although the dollar amounts are staggering, it hardly touches on the emotional and spiritual costs of addiction—the lost and wasted human potential, the devastation to families and communities.

One factor that bears constant repeating is that young people are much more susceptible to becoming addicted—the young brain is supremely vulnerable to this disease. Califano writes that for more than a decade, 12 to 17 year olds have named drugs as the number-one problem they face when responding to an open-ended question in the annual back-to-school survey of the National Center on Addiction and Substance Abuse (CASA) at Columbia University. As Califano points out, if you can keep individuals off drugs, cigarettes, and alcohol until they reach adulthood, the chances of them becoming addicted diminish almost to the point that it is no longer a threat.

I bring this up not only because it gives us more insight into the beginnings of this disease, but also because it should be shouted from rooftops across the land that there is a moral imperative to protect the young from the devastating effects of addictive substances. In all my years of listening to addicts and their stories, I cannot recall one story where the using did not begin when the addicted were in their youth. There of course may be exceptions, but this is a powerfully tragic truth and a strong indictment against those who would sell and market these life-destroying substances to the young. Again, it is not enough to tell young people what not to do; we must also tell them and model what *to* do; this is the great hope and challenge of Integral Recovery.

So, why *another* book on recovery? A great and valid question. The answer is that by using the Integral map, developed by Ken Wilber,[6] a philosopher of extraordinary breadth, depth, and erudition, and other Integral pioneers, we can look at the disease of addiction with new eyes and a new understanding that has never before been available to us. The Integral map enables us to avoid making the crucial mistake of neglecting key aspects of the addictive process and allows us to cover all the essential bases. Viewing the disease of addiction through the lens of the Integral map is what separates Integral Recovery from other holistic approaches to treatment.

The problem with prior models lies not in how they deal with some of the important aspects of the disease, but that they lack a means to deal with *all* the vital aspects of addiction. In Integral thought, we say that "everyone is right in what they affirm but err in what they neglect." Because addiction affects and eventually destroys the addicted person comprehensively, in all the fundamental dimensions of his or her life, it is vital that all the affected and infected parts be addressed, understood, and healed. If we leave any holes in the dike, it will not hold back the ocean over time, and if we leave a big hole or many holes, the dike will collapse quickly, and those whom the dike was intended to protect will be swept away.

For example, while Alcoholics Anonymous includes great community support and inspiration, as well as acknowledging and working on the spiritual aspects of the disease, it does not include the latest neurological and genetic science, which has a huge part to play in healing the disease of addiction. And, even the most cutting-edge, holistic approaches to addiction, which do endeavor to include the body, mind, heart, and soul, do not include developmental stages or types, which, when used within an Integral framework, effect an absolute quantum leap in our understanding and approach to treatment.

What Is Integral Recovery?

I am often asked, What exactly is "Integral"? And, What does it mean when you use it in the title *Integral Recovery*? I hope that this book will clarify exactly what Integral means in relation to recovery, but I will offer a simple explanation from the start. Integral is holism with a map. Let me explain. Take the example of traditional medicine. Many of us, over the years, have come to realize that traditional medicine, while very effective in so many ways, completely misses the boat in many other very important ways (addiction for example). We have rightly seen and intuited that standard allopathic medicine seems to have emerged in a vacuum, often treating its patients as if they, too, had developed in a vacuum, where physical bodies are divorced from minds, spirits, relations, nutrition, cultures, and the world around us. The physicians and those of us who advocate for consideration of these things, when treating a patient, are kept outside the circle of acceptable "true medicine" and are thought to have moved into the realm of the fanciful and unscientific, even when our holistic leanings are totally in congruence with the leading edge of many fields of science.

Holism is an emergent way of viewing the world that was largely brought into the modern and now postmodern West, by the mind-blowing and paradigm-shattering findings in the field of quantum mechanics and quantum physics: Time is relative. Matter is energy. The observer affects the observed. Goodbye objective science and our firm grasp on the nature of reality![7]

The psychedelic sixties also helped many of us deconstruct our divided and subdivided universe; in our psychedelic visions, we could clearly see that we were split within ourselves and separate from each other, the earth, and nature. Most of our academic disciplines and sciences would not even talk to each other. Of course, developmentally, there is a time when separation and autonomy are beneficial—for example, when science was let loose to advance on its own, rather than forced through the ecclesiastical filter of the Bible. As soon as science became unfettered and unthreatened by religion, the modern world could be born. But by the middle of the twentieth century, we had moved beyond the point where an atomistic and autonomous view of the world was useful. What had formerly been the way out became the trap. Humpty Dumpty had taken a great and useful fall, but now the task was how to put him back together again. How could so many diverse and beautiful pieces be reunited in a life-enhancing, world-restoring, unitive vision and practice?

The holistic intuition was that individual parts cannot be comprehended or treated effectively if they are not understood as part of a larger whole. The sum of the parts creates a greater whole, and the parts themselves are without meaning if placed into a vacuum. Try to imagine a human being with nothing else. It's impossible! The holistic quest became to re-member the world and re-member our essential unity, so that we cease to act in unwise and harmful ways. The hope was that perhaps by bringing all these parts back together, we could create a better world and a better future for ourselves, our children, and all life forms.

Presently, the word "holistic" has been used so much that it has become somewhat of a cliché: there are so many versions of holistic, each one interpreted by someone claiming to be holistic in his approach and practice, that the word often loses its meaning. In the world of wilderness therapy (my field of endeavor for a couple of decades), the word holistic is all the rage when describing new programs. What it generally means is that a program may pay more attention to diet than in the past, and perhaps throw in some yoga and meditation (or something along these lines). I myself have struggled while developing programs, knowing that traditional treatment methods were missing big pieces of the puzzle and wondering if my model managed to include all that was necessary and essential for recovering the health of my students.

When I co-founded Passages to Recovery, a therapeutic wilderness program for adults suffering from alcoholism and other forms of addiction,[8] I could see how previous wilderness models had left out major areas that needed attention if our students were to have a better chance of getting well and staying sober. So I studied the brain, nutrition, meditation, yoga, and any other fields of knowledge I thought would be useful and tried to put them all together in a new and creative way. It was pretty good, sort of like being an intuitive cook: add a little of this and a little of that, put it on the stove, and hopefully it will turn out not only edible but also tasting good. This is how the holistic approach developed: body, mind, spirit, nature, and yeah! Let's see what we can do. It wasn't very clear and rightly criticized as being rather mushy and murky. So, while intuiting and understanding that a holistic approach was necessary and superior, I struggled with how to identify all that was necessary to consider and how to fit it all together.

Then, in 2004, when I read a paper by Ken Wilber that was published on the internet,[9] in which he described the Integral (or AQAL[10]) map, I immediately understood that this was the map that the emerging holistic world view needed to become radically more holistic and hence effective. It included the essential dimensions of reality (the four quadrants), multiple human intelligences (lines), stages of growth (developmental maps), states of consciousness, and typologies, with a clear understanding that we had to deal with our personal and collective shadows and that the way to bring this understanding beautifully into fruition—into our world, our lives, and our bodies—was through dedicated, ongoing Integral practices. The more I looked at it, the more I saw.[11]

The Integral map shows us all that is absolutely essential for us to consider on every occasion and also how it all fits together.[12] The map is what makes the Integral approach both revolutionary and powerful. In our times of increasing complexity, this map serves as an operating system that allows us to organize information and integrate it in ways that were unimaginable in the past. The Integral map enables us to embrace complexity and change, whether in the life of an individual or concerning any issue, challenge, or problem—in our case the treatment of addiction—rather than throwing up our hands in despair or retreating to simplistic solutions that don't work because essential dimensions are being neglected or left out. The Integral map takes holism from a brilliant intuition to a brilliant blueprint, and Integral practice takes the brilliant blueprint into life-changing, multidimensional reality.

A short definition of Integral Recovery is a lifetime Integral Recovery Practice illuminated by the Integral map. *Integral Recovery Practice,* at the core of Integral Recovery, is a sophisticated system of personal development that engages body, mind, heart, and spirit in daily practices designed to produce extraordinary health and awakening on all levels of our being. I will introduce these essential practices in the second half of the book; as the chapter headings denote, the focus is on building the body, transforming the brain, healing the emotions, the power of transmuting the shadow, and healing the spirit. Maintaining the practices with ongoing, lifelong dedication is the key to mastering a life of recovery.

The framework offered by the Integral approach to recovery from addiction is self-correcting in that it expects, encourages, and integrates change and evolution of the model itself as new information, data, and modalities emerge and come online. The model will become more effective, more elegant, and more beautiful as it evolves and grows. I make no claims that Integral Recovery is a cure for addiction—it is not a magic bullet—but each part of the map, each practice, and each insight is a nudge in the right direction. And as these many nudges accumulate and synergize each other, soon we find that we are nudged right off the board and into an entirely new game altogether: the disease of addiction has become the adventure of creating our highest and best selves.

Here are just a few of the benefits of the Integral Recovery approach to treating addiction:

1. It's a much more encouraging and attractive model than those currently in use, as the emphasis is on personal growth, not just the negativity of addiction. The focus is not merely on "not using," but on emotional, intellectual, and spiritual growth and physical well-being.

2. It transcends the traditional dichotomy of "addict" and "non-addict." In the Integral Recovery approach, everyone is a practitioner, including the treatment provider.

3. It offers a more complete accounting of the causes of addiction, and therefore it points the way as to how one can address those causes.

4. It features a deeper understanding of the internal mechanisms of healing, growth, and transcendence and how they relate to the recovering individual.

5. It provides a framework with which to rationally examine and judiciously use a variety of treatment approaches, uniting multiple partial modalities into an integrated whole.

6. It supplies skillful treatment and relapse prevention, teaching an individualized Integral Recovery Practice as the fundamental vehicle of the recovery process.

7. It presents a comprehensive and detailed map of the journey of recovery—one that's inspiring, enlightening, and immediately practical.

The Integral model represents the cutting edge of thinking on the integration of science, spirituality, and human development, presenting a conceptual framework that allows many different schools of thought to meaningfully and usefully coexist and at the same time inform and enrich each other. The Integral map not only enables us to understand the problem of addiction and how best to approach it, but perhaps even more importantly, it helps us understand ourselves and our place in the world. It illuminates the journey of recovery in comprehensive and compassionate terms. In teaching this model to adolescents, I have seen the scales fall from their eyes as they begin to understand and put it together. They often say, "Why hasn't anyone told us this before?" I answer, "Because until very recently, nobody knew it."

Christian theologian Matthew Fox[13] has written that in a culture where young people are not given any method for transcendence, substance abuse and addiction are assured. A method of transcendence is exactly what the Integral map and an Integral Recovery Practice *do* offer us; Integral Recovery is an antidote not only for addiction, but also for the cultural soil that nourishes the disease. The Integral map is illuminating and inspiring and, in my experience, generally finds immediate resonance in the minds of health care professionals as well as those suffering from the disease of addiction and their families.

Having been a professional wilderness guide for many years, I know the need for good maps. As this book unfolds, we will explore what an Integral approach looks like, and how it can dramatically improve our understanding of addiction and vastly improve the successful outcome of treatment, moving beyond mere sobriety to a lifelong journey of optimal health, self-actualization, and ultimately Self-realization. But first, here is how I arrived at this Integral approach to recovery.

My Life: The Short Version

As a baby boomer, I was born into an era where alcohol use and smoking tobacco were socially accepted norms, at least in the professional, upwardly mobile circles my family moved in. Alcohol was used in my home, but never apparently abused, and I can find no instance of alcoholism in my genetic makeup. However, drinking was part of the cultural landscape of both my parents' worlds, Cajun Catholic on my father's side and Mississippi Scotch Irish WASP on my mother's side.

Enter the sixties. My first experience of illegal drugs was through my older brother, who was an early hippie and was experimenting with marijuana and psychedelics by 1967. He told me enthusiastically about his experiences, and on occasion, I witnessed him under the influence. I personally was caught up in the brilliant, drug-catalyzed music of the late sixties—the Beatles, Jimi Hendrix, Bob Dylan, Cream, and the Doors were some of my favorites. I began experimenting with pot and psychedelics when I was 13. I was attracted to the transcendental and idealistic aspects of the counterculture, including the altered states of consciousness that could be experienced with drugs.

Early in 1970, however, I began to notice the changing nature of the drug scene where I lived; peace and love were turning into greed

and paranoia. I lost my best friend over this shift, as he became seriously hooked on heroin. I was struggling with my own use, looking for
some kind of spiritual clarity and intuiting that something had gone very
wrong and that somehow drugs were not doing it—whatever "it" was.

That summer, I dropped out of the drug world and embarked on
an eight-year journey into radical, evangelical, counterculture Christianity. Eight years later, I found myself sober, disillusioned, and directionally
clueless. I joined the army, became a military police investigator in Ger-
many, and found myself on the law enforcement side of the illegal drug
problem. To me, the issue appeared cut and dried: There are rules. If you
break the rules, you need to pay the price. Besides, I thought, protecting
free Western Europe from the Soviet juggernaut was important. I didn't
think being messed up on drugs was mission-friendly. Morally, the issues
seemed clear to me, but I was not blind to the suffering of the addicted
soldiers I busted and interrogated in the course of my investigations.

After my discharge, I went to college. It was 1982. Cocaine was king.
In the course of things, I tried cocaine twice. I loved it. Some deeper,
wiser part of me said, "You can never do this again." I listened, and I
didn't. I did fall in love with a young woman who was dependent on
marijuana and saw how she smoked not to get high, but to feel normal;
when the pot ran out, there was anxiety and chaos. The popular thinking
at the time, and even now, was that pot was not addictive. It clearly was.
In short, I was coming to see drug abuse and addiction from another
perspective.

My first job out of college was as a counselor at a residential
wilderness program in East Texas, the Salesmanship Club Boy's Camp. I
worked with a group of 12, 13, and 14 year olds in an isolated part of
the woods in structures we built ourselves. In the woods with the boys
and my co-counselors, I found something very important for an idealistic
young man: direction. My inner compass started pointing at a rather foggy
north. I began to see rather vague signs that read "spirituality . . . healing . . . wilderness." As nebulous as this might seem, here was something
that I could give my life to—something of value.

This led to my traveling to the San Francisco Bay area and enroll-
ing at John F. Kennedy University to study Transpersonal Psychology. I
learned a lot about spirituality, some about psychology, made some good
friends, and met the woman who would later become my wife and life
companion. But I learned virtually nothing about addiction or chemical
dependency. I later found out this was commonly true of almost all of the

graduate psychology programs at the time, not to mention the medical schools. Fortunately, there are some signs that this may be changing. Psychology and medical students are now beginning to learn a bit about the disease of addiction, but it's still not much, and it's definitely not enough.

During this period, I worked at an adolescent treatment center in Oakland called Thunder Road. This was real work, in the trenches, with teens of all ethnic and socioeconomic backgrounds. I learned the Twelve Steps of Alcoholics Anonymous, taught them, ran groups, had an individual caseload, and worked with the families. I was delighted that the AA model allowed us to talk about spiritual matters, and I was amazed to see beautiful people emerge from their angry, self-centered, addictive spell. I attended dozens of AA meetings with my clients and listened to many stories of drug abuse, addiction, and despair. But I felt terrible fear when my clients graduated and went back to their lives. Many of them had accomplished coming out of their drug-induced haze, healing, and getting the first inklings of something spiritual, but I knew that for most of them, the traditional injunction to attend 90 meetings in 90 days, get a sponsor, and work the steps, was not going to see them all the way through to a successful recovery.

After eight years in the Bay Area, I heard the call of the wild again and moved with my partner to the Southern Utah desert. We spent six months knocking around in an old four-wheel-drive truck—exploring, hiking, learning about the animals, plants, geology, and history, and vision questing. It was a very rich time with new vistas of beauty and revelation seemingly behind every turn in the road and bend in the canyon. Eventually, our wanderings brought us to an outdoor wilderness therapy program for adolescents, the Aspen Achievement Academy in Loa, Utah. It was mutual love at first sight, and we were hired on the spot. That was 1994.

The next decade was dedicated, for the most part, to wilderness therapy. During that time, I worked with hundreds of students and their families. The underlying problems for most of the students were the old nemeses: drug abuse, alcoholism, and addiction. There is no doubt in my mind that therapeutic wilderness programs can be a powerful clinical intervention and that most of the people in the industry are skillful, caring, intelligent people with the highest motivations. But wilderness does not cure addiction. What it does do is temporarily break the ever-downward-spiraling addictive cycle, at least for a time, giving both students and their families time to regroup and consider their options.

The problem I began to look at was what happens when the program is over. Sending students back to their old stomping grounds almost never works if they are addicts. For most, the old playgrounds and playmates are overwhelming relapse triggers. The more money the family has, the greater the options, and the standard aftercare plan among those with the means consists of sending the afflicted student to a therapeutic boarding school of some sort until they are eighteen, keeping them safe, and hoping for the best. Sometimes this works; sometimes it doesn't. If addicts want drugs, they will find a way to get them. You could send an addict to a penal colony in Siberia, and if he wanted to, he would still manage to get high.

In the late nineties, I began working on an idea for a new type of wilderness program, one that would face the beast of addiction eye to eye, instead of treating it as a secondary concern. I was given the opportunity to build such a program under the corporate aegis of the Aspen Education Group, the parent company that owned Aspen Achievement Academy, my original employer in Utah. On January 15, 2001, I had built my team and gathered my first group of students. We wandered for a month in the San Rafael Desert in Southern Utah, most of the time in heavy snow and subfreezing weather. The results were exhilarating. We had taken a group of seven ne'er–do–well alcoholics, addicts, and thugs from New Jersey and hiked hundreds of miles in an isolated, freezing desert; we had meditated, sweated, prayed, told our stories, and worked the Twelve Steps; and we had culminated the experience with a vision quest. We had deeply bonded as a group, and almost every person had experienced a moral and spiritual awakening.

This was so impressive that it was decided we should continue the project; this program became Passages to Recovery. We attracted an exceptional staff who were inspired by the blatantly spiritual nature of our program. I also spent a lot of time attempting to hire recovery "experts," but I soon found out that what passes for an expert in the field of recovery is normally an alcoholic or addict who has a respectable amount of sober time. This is a helpful perspective; however, it is limited in determining an individual's skills or qualifications to counsel, teach, and lead recovering addicts though the wilderness.[14]

Having a hard time finding the experts I sought, I set out to make myself one. I read, researched, and built a personal recovery and treatment library. I listened to story after story of people afflicted with the disease, both in and out of our program. I studied the *Big Book* of AA and other AA literature. I worked the Twelve Steps. I developed and wrote a curriculum for Passages and taught it to our staff and students. I became known as "John, the recovery expert." I found this somewhat ironic and amusing, but I stepped into the role.

As inspiring and powerful as Passages to Recovery was, I soon discovered it was not enough. The problem with Passages—and all treatment centers, no matter how good they are, or how poor for that matter—is that eventually the patient has to leave. In the case of Passages, our students would often leave positively radiant in a glow of inspiration and new hope for their lives. However, in many cases, this light would soon fade, and we were acutely aware of this.

Two courses of action typically recommended for students leaving a program were either, 1. Go to a secondary treatment center, where you can further your education or get a job; where there will indeed be opportunities for relapse to occur, but at the same time you will have support around learning to live a sober life. (Yet in this case, you will eventually have to leave the secondary center and return to the world.) Or, 2. The traditional possibility was to leave the program, find an AA or an NA meeting, get a sponsor, work the steps, eventually become a sponsor, and continue working the program for the rest of your life. This sometimes works, but not often enough.

The idea has often been that it is not AA or the program that is flawed, but you. It works if you work it, etc. Well, that idea didn't work for me. Something was terribly amiss; more was needed. I had some vague ideas but couldn't quite put it together. As time went on, I took the whole thing very personally, exhausted myself, and fell into a deep depression. I was not alone. Exhaustion and burnout are all too common among those laboring on the front line in this field.

Enter Integral. At some point in 2004, I was browsing through the magazine *The Utne Reader* and saw an advertisement for a website[15] that mentioned Ken Wilber and a host of other luminaries, whose books I had read or at least heard of. I checked it out, signed up for a month's free membership, and read a forty-page PDF file by Ken Wilber called "Introduction to Integral Theory and Practice: The AQAL Map."[16] The more I read, the more excited I became. My discouraged, fragmented, and exhausted mind opened with tremendous clarity. "This is it!" I thought. Here, in Integral theory, were the missing ingredients, the organizing principles that had been lacking in the recovery field.

I was completely captivated and spent the next couple of months looking for the Integral authority who was applying the AQAL map to the treatment of addiction. After a couple of months, the sobering (pun intended) notion dawned on me that no one was doing this yet and that perhaps I was the guy who needed to step up to the plate. I had no idea of the extent of the journey I was about to embark on. What started as an attempt to find a better way of treating addiction also became a personal journey of renewal and self-transformation. What follows is what I have found so far on this journey. This is not to be the last word on Integral Recovery, but the first.

1

Recovery from What?

The Disease of Addiction

When the *Big Book* of Alcoholics Anonymous was published in 1939,[1] the neurological basis of addiction was completely unknown. In a foreword to the *Big Book*, there is a brief chapter titled "The Doctor's Opinion," in which the writer, Dr. William Silkworth, describes alcoholism as an allergy. This conclusion was based upon years of working with alcoholics and looking at alcoholism from an outside, third-person perspective. This seemed to fit the facts as they were then known: some people drink, and they are fine; and some people drink, and they are possessed by booze, eventually drinking themselves to death.

Identifying alcoholism as an allergy was a plausible explanation. Unfortunately, this medical explanation did not catch on. Despite the proposition that addiction could be seen as an objective, physical problem—one that, presumably, could be treated through medical means the notion persisted that addiction must be some kind of moral and ethical deficiency and not the purview of medicine. Doctors washed their hands of the whole messy issue and shifted responsibility for the problem to law enforcement. This has caused a health care catastrophe. It does not mean that law enforcement has no role to play in an overall Integral approach. But, first and foremost, we must realize that addiction is not a crime but a disease. Let me state it clearly at the beginning of our discussion: addiction is a disease of the brain, which involves relapse and requires a lifetime strategy of ongoing practice and care. I would like to note here that I am not attached to the idea that a lifetime of care and treatment will always be the only answer to addiction. But the word "cure" is tossed around a lot these days in the context of addiction, and I do not believe that it is accurate or helpful to use it.

15

Let's diverge for a moment and consider a better understood disease: type 1 diabetes. The organ affected is the pancreas. The defect is that the organ is no longer producing sufficient insulin. Some of the symptoms are excessive thirst, extreme hunger, unusual weight loss, increased weight, irritability, and blurred vision. Left untreated, diabetes results in death. With treatment, which includes insulin injections and appropriate diet, the symptoms disappear, and the diabetic can begin to live a normal and productive life. As far as I know, there is no Diabetics Anonymous. Anonymity is not necessary when there is no social stigma associated with the disease.

Let us look at addiction in the same light. The organ is the brain. The defect is the brain's inability to produce sufficient dopamine and other essential neurochemicals. The symptoms are uncontrollable cravings for the drug of choice, and the behaviors that accompany these overpowering cravings are, among others, lying, stealing, radical negative personality changes (which I call the Dr. Jekyll/Mr. Hyde syndrome), and withdrawal from formerly important relationships. Looking at these behaviors, the assumption has been that addicts are "bad" people and have what has been popularly called an "addictive personality." This interpretation has been further reinforced by the fact that approximately 80 percent of our 1.8 million prison population is incarcerated on drug- and alcohol-related charges or crimes that stem directly from addiction, including the use and sale of these substances.[2]

A further challenge presented by addiction, as well as by other brain diseases such as schizophrenia and depression, is that there has been no objective test for diagnosis. Instead, all we have to go on is first looking at the behaviors and then listening to the patients' subjective descriptions of their experiences, along with subjective reports from family or friends.

So we say addiction is a brain disease, but how do we know this? Our first knowledge came as a result of the famous Olds experiments in the 1950s, when Olds set out to find the locus of addiction in the brain.[3] As often happens, the first experimental subjects were rats. Rats, like humans, have a triune brain (albeit in the case of the rat, much less sophisticated than its human counterpart), whose main parts are the cortex, the limbic system, and the midbrain, sometimes called the reptilian stem. These three layers contain our evolutionary neurological history and inheritance. The neo or frontal cortex governs the higher human functions such as love, meaning, values, and spirituality. The limbic system deals with emotions, and the midbrain, or reptilian stem, with very powerful, primitive survival instincts, such as killing, eating, and reproductive urges.

Since the addict (in the mid to latter stages of the disease) seems to lose touch with the higher human functions and values, it was assumed, quite logically, that the problem had to be in the neocortex. So Olds and colleagues injected cocaine into the brain of a rat—expecting that the behaviors associated with cocaine use and addiction would rapidly manifest. What happened? Zip. They continued this line of research throughout the cortex, thinking they had maybe missed a spot; again, nothing. Olds and his colleagues then proceeded through the limbic system—again with no results.

Finally, as we might imagine, a bit discouraged, they tried the earliest and least suspect part of the brain, the midbrain. Eureka! They had it. The rats exhibited many of the behaviors associated with cocaine use and, quickly, addiction. The rats were given a lever with which they could self-regulate injections of cocaine into their midbrains, and they simply continued to hit the lever until they starved to death. (Is this starting to sound familiar?) Then the scientists experimented with sending increasing voltages of electricity through the floor on which the rats had to stand in order to move the cocaine-injecting lever, and the rats went right on hitting the lever until they were electrocuted.

The conclusion? The first part of the brain that is taken over and altered by the disease is the midbrain, which controls our most primitive and basic survival instincts. In short order, this hijacking will change the form and function of other parts of the brain as well.[4] But already, in the brain of the addict, addictive cravings have become equated with survival—not pleasure, not fun, but survival. Incessant cravings for drugs have become so primary that all other instincts and drives are secondary in importance. Eventually the cravings become more powerful than the instinct for life itself.

What these experiments with rats show us is that addiction has nothing to do with character defects, moral failings, or sin. I doubt theologians would agree that it is possible for a rat to sin, but it is clear that rats can, and do, become addicts. Behaviorally, this is all very perplexing, but neurobiologically, when looking at the brain, it is very simple.

In a healthy brain, successful accomplishment of essential survival activities controlled by the midbrain, such as hunting, eating, and sex, is rewarded with a pleasurable surge of dopamine. This neurochemical produces the rush, the thrill, the sense of "Yes!" (This certainly explains our attraction to war, violence, and contact sports.) The surge of dopamine is then followed by a surge of serotonin, a neurochemical that produces an experience of satiation and satisfaction, which balances out the dopamine.

However, in the brain of the addict, this natural reward system is hijacked; naturally occurring and necessary survival behaviors no longer produce pleasurable feelings. This is because our drug use has quickly exhausted and depleted our natural supplies of dopamine and serotonin, so, we, as addicts, can no longer feel pleasure and satisfaction *without the addictive substance* (which serves as artificial dopamine). In the absence of the drug, and with virtually no serotonin and dopamine supplies left, the brain kicks in large amounts of norepinephrine, the brain's adrenaline, which causes the addict to suffer anxiety, the shakes, and sweating—otherwise known as symptoms of withdrawal.

As the brain continues to reduce the number of dopamine receptors in response to the flooding of the brain with pseudo dopamine (drugs), the addict must take ever greater quantities in an attempt to achieve the same effects. This is known as tolerance. One sees this reflected in the using patterns of late-stage addicts, when they are able to consume mass amounts of drugs that would normally kill a horse. A slight exception is found in the latter stages of the alcoholic's disease, when the alcohol begins to destroy the liver. At that point, it takes very little alcohol to achieve the desired effect. A particularly dangerous aspect of tolerance, in the specific case of heroin addicts, is that as the heroin addict detoxes, the brain begins to try and heal itself, causing more dopamine receptors to come back online. If the heroin addict then leaves treatment, relapses, and attempts to use the same dosage he was formerly using, he often overdoses and dies, not realizing that his tolerance had been significantly decreased during detox and his time of abstinence from using drugs.

Brain chemistry in the "addictive personality" can also be changed with behaviors besides drugs. A person who is identified as having an addictive personality might be one who falls into a series of compulsive behaviors involving, for example, sex, video games, food addictions, internet pornography, exercise, shopping, or gambling—all of which are attempts to alter their brain chemistry in order to feel "okay." A person with a healthy, balanced brain can make choices about pleasurable activities, whereas the person with neurochemical imbalances feels constant anxiety, depression, or dissatisfaction. The use of different activities to try to feel better then leads to a reliance on the activities that is compulsive. Now the activities are no longer freely chosen, but acted out in a trance-like and robotic manner, and they lead not to satiation and satisfaction, but to progressively stronger cravings and suffering. So what looks to the outside observer like a personality or character issue is actually the outward manifestation of a neurological disorder.

When addicts suffer cravings, these are not like a nonaddicted person's cravings for a good meal, or a new car, but cravings so powerful that in the brain they are equated with existence and survival. It's not, "I sure would like . . . ," but "I've got to have!" The locus of control is no longer the moral, caring neocortex, but the powerful, primitive reptilian brain. In a psychologically healthy situation, our higher self controls our lower drives. In the addict's brain, this is turned upside down. This explains perfectly the addict's bad behaviors: the lying, the stealing, the manipulative use of others, and the radical negative personality changes. The more highly evolved cortex becomes the slave of the reptilian midbrain and its overpowering, "gotta have it," compulsively perceived survival needs.

Am I an Addict?

Why are some people addicts and others not? We are not sure, but it seems that 10 percent of us have the propensity to become addicted.[5] I would venture to say that it is rare in our society when a young person gets through high school and college without some contact with potentially addictive substances. This is unfortunate, because studies[6] tell us that if young people can make it to adulthood without using alcohol, drugs, or tobacco, the chances of their becoming addicted are virtually nil—or, if not nil, greatly decreased. In any case, a lot of us move through these years, experimenting, partying, and in some cases abusing, but we don't become hooked; we stop altogether or moderate to some level that works for us in a reasonable way.

In one of the initial talks I give to students in treatment, titled "Am I an Addict?" I make it clear from the outset that I have no agenda to prove somebody *is* an addict; I simply want to conduct an inquiry, consider the facts, examine the symptoms, and allow people to make an honest self-diagnosis. If you dissect your own experience using the following three characteristics of addiction, it's usually very clear whether you are an addict or not, and to what degree.

1. Addiction Is Progressive

It starts out as a small thing, seemingly harmless, like a minor cut or a localized infection. But with time, if left untreated, it spreads throughout the body and eventually kills the patient. This means that in the initial phases of the disease, it is often difficult to tell whether one is clinically addicted or merely abusing a substance. It's important to remember that not everyone who uses or even abuses is necessarily addicted, and in the early stages of the disease abusers and addicts look very much the same. But as the disease progresses to its later stages, it becomes obvious to an informed person what is going on, and eventually it becomes clear to the addict himself. The first key to understanding the disease is that it is progressive. Addiction starts out as a small thing and progresses into a huge, uncontrollable thing.

What distinguishes the addict from the abuser? It's just this: at some point the abuser gets sick and tired of the negative consequences of his abuse and makes a decision to quit or moderate his use—and does. For addicts, this is virtually impossible. They see and recognize the negative consequences of their use (at least some part of them does), but they have lost the capacity to control the intake of the substance. When working with late-stage clients, I often ask the question, "What do you think about 24/7, from the time you get up until the time you pass out?" Usually, this will lead to an "Aha!" moment of self-recognition. The answer, of course, is drugs and/or drinking. The cravings and the urge to use or drink have become all consuming.

Often there is an initial phase of the disease that I call the "romance phase," when the addict discovers the substance or substances, and it is as if he has found the answer to all of his problems. "I don't have to be sad anymore. I don't have to be shy or depressed. I don't have to feel unattractive or uncool. This is wonderful!" As you might imagine, this phase of the disease is hard to treat. Why? Because, normally, the last thing on earth that the addict wants to do at this point is stop using— the drug(s) is meeting so many needs. This can involve, for example, a new peer group and social acceptance within that circle or a new profession, which often entails dealing drugs or otherwise carrying out illegal or objectionable actions in order to support one's habit. In fact, a whole new life can open up, which seems very appealing at first but then changes over time to become a complete hell.[7] Feeling peace or even feeling ecstatic for the first time in one's life is very powerful. While relating their first experience of using their favorite drug, many addicts have described it to me as love at first swallow, snort, or fix. The addict, in short, has fallen in love.

A teacher of mine once looked into my eyes and told me, "You have some good pain in you." What he was saying was that I had suffered deeply enough that I might get real and get down to work on myself.

This is often the case with addicts. Frequently, they have to become sick of their relationship with the drug and its consequences before they can begin to do the hard work of healing. In AA parlance, this is known as "hitting bottom" and is generally seen as a necessary condition for beginning the day-to-day work of returning to health. All too often, an addict will come to a meeting and say, "I can control my drinking." The response is, "Okay, go and try some controlled drinking." The alcoholic eventually returns after much suffering, not at all in control of her drinking, and admits that she has lost the ability to control her drinking (the first step of AA). Then the work begins.

There is a certain validity to this concept, but it is not acceptable if one is a parent and the idea is, Oh, wait until your teenage daughter is selling her body to get drugs—then we can intervene. Absolutely not! One does not have to wait until someone destroys his or her life before one acts. In the recovery industry, this is called "raising the bottom." (A former student of mine recently quipped, "You hit bottom where you stop digging.") There are plenty of external motivators that can be, and usually must be, put into place to supply the necessary incentives to get and stay sober.

The overwhelming majority of people who enter treatment are not there because they want to be, but because they have to be. Each stage of the disease, the romance stage, the balancing act stage (where the addict is still trying to maintain some semblance of normalcy), and the over-the-edge stage (when the addict has stopped even trying to fool himself—when it's just all about taking drugs) is treatable, but each stage presents its own challenges. It is interesting to note that success rates in treatment seem to be the same for those who enter voluntarily and those who enter treatment through the use of external motivators such as the threat of jail time or the loss of their job, marriage, or financial support.[8] I have seen everything from "F___ you, I don't want to be here," to a young man sobbing in my arms the second day of treatment saying, "I can't use heroin again. If I do, I'm going to put a pistol in my mouth and pull the trigger." He knew that heroin was killing him (in fact it had killed his father), but he felt powerless to stop. Self-annihilation looked like a better alternative than further descent into the maelstrom of heroin addiction.

Another interesting aspect of the progression of the disease is that one's addiction seems to become more powerful, even during periods of abstinence. I have often observed this phenomenon: a person will enter treatment, clean up, restore some degree of her health, leave treatment, stay sober for a while, and then suddenly relapse. Many times the addict will tell herself: "This time it will be different. Now that I've worked on some of my issues, and I'm healthier and stronger, I will be able to handle it." Not only does this *not* happen, but instead of picking up where she left off, the addict self now seems to want to make up for lost time. She uses more than before she went into treatment! Why is this so? We don't know, but, based on many years of experience and reams of anecdotal evidence, this appears to be the case. There does seem to be a consensus emerging that if the original complaints or sufferings that started the person using and self-medicating in the first place are addressed on emotional, spiritual, physical, neurobiological, and even cellular levels, then this sort of relapse does not have to occur. This is the bright promise of the future as we begin to move from treatment to cure.

2. Addiction Is Chronic

Once you have crossed the line from use to addiction, there is no going back. Addiction doesn't just get up and go away. It is not just a phase, and one does not outgrow it. As Bill Wilson wrote in the *Big Book* of Alcoholics Anonymous, it is the dream of every alcoholic to be able to drink like a normal person. Unfortunately, the alcoholic relates to his drinking in a completely different way than the "normal" person. For example, an alcoholic seated in a restaurant who sees someone leaving half a glass of wine unfinished will simply, viscerally, not be able to understand how this is possible. Likewise, the nonalcoholic will not comprehend how the alcoholic can't stop drinking when he is staggeringly drunk and his life, health, and relationships are collapsing all around him because of his drinking.

The fact is that once you're addicted, you don't become unaddicted. This means you can never safely use the addictive substances again. This also means that if you were addicted to heroin, for example, it's not okay for you to drink alcohol or smoke pot. All of these drugs affect the same part of the brain and can trigger the same renewed, virtually uncontrollable cravings.

As our understanding of addiction continues to grow, let me make this clarification. Up until very recently, most recovery experts spoke of chemical dependency synonymously with addiction. Presently, a new understanding is emerging that one can become chemically dependent without becoming an addict. An example of this would be if an individual was in a traumatic accident and had injuries so severe as to require powerful narcotics to treat the pain. After a few weeks of using these drugs, the individual decides, or his physician decides, it's time to quit. By that time, the individual has become chemically dependent on these drugs. When he quits, he experiences all the symptoms of withdrawal from an addictive substance. However, after that, it's over. He never craves these substances again. That is chemical dependency without addiction.

In the case of the addict, however, one could be separated from her drug of choice, alcohol, for example, for years, maybe in prison, and when she is released, the cravings that have never left her take over again, and she is right back where she was, or quickly even lower than before. This is an addict. What we're finding is that the brain of the addict has been changed in its function by the disease of addiction. We can actually see the change in the function of the brain through CAT scans and other brain imaging technologies.

The Dr. Jekyll/Mr. Hyde Syndrome

The "Dr. Jekyll/Mr. Hyde syndrome" describes the radical personality change that happens to the addict as the disease takes its course. The formerly good, kind Dr. Jekyll transforms into the monstrous Mr. Hyde. This is not a loose literary parallel. Robert Louis Stevenson was actually writing a metaphorical story about the effects of cocaine. The once loving son, daughter, husband, wife, mother, father, friend, or other loved one turns into a raging, manipulative, self-centered addict. The change is dramatic and horrifying.[9]

Periodically, the healthy self will reemerge, feel great remorse for her behaviors, and promise to quit using and change. This is sincerely felt by the individual. But this is no longer possible without treatment and outside help. The addict self comes back, sooner or later, and those close to the addict experience it as another betrayal, which, in fact, it is. The addict realizes this also, which only adds to the shame and despair, fueling renewed use and self-narcotization.

3. Addiction Is Terminal

The last point is that the condition is terminal; if not treated, the patient dies. What we are treating is the progressive, uncontrollable compulsion to use drugs, which, if unchecked, leads finally to death (and/or in many cases incarceration). This does not mean there aren't what we call "functional drunks," addicts who can muddle through life and hold it together for years, and some who can even accomplish great things, such as Ernest Hemingway, Henry the VIII, Jack Kerouac, Trungpa Rinpoche, and so on. Often these are very creative people, but if one looks at the quality of their interpersonal relationships and their ultimate demise, one can clearly see the footprints of the disease, subtle at first, and eventually grinding them into the ground.

The Villains of the Story: Causes of Addiction

Whether we become addicts or not is often largely a matter of genetics and the newly emerging field of epigenetics. If a person has a grandparent that is an alcoholic, there is a four times greater chance that he will also become addicted. If both parents are addicted, the chances are eight times greater. Also, some ethnic groups are apparently more susceptible than others. For example, among the Cherokee there is almost no chance of using alcohol and not becoming addicted. In my work with students in recovery programs, one of my first questions is, "Is there a history of alcoholism or addiction in your biological family?" The response is almost always 100 percent, "Yes."

While genetics seem to play a very important role, not every person who has the genetic potential becomes addicted. In most cases, genes seem to be a necessary factor but not a sufficient causal factor. What is the other factor that triggers the genetic potential for addiction? Stress. Let me state that again. *Stress.* Chronic, inescapable, unavoidable stress is public enemy number one in the brain of those who possess the genetic potential for addiction. This is a good reason treatment should not be punitive; treatment involves healing and rebalancing the brain and learning to have pleasure in natural, drug-free ways. Being punitive, however, only causes stress in the individual, hence renewed cravings and then relapse.

Stress that happens early and stress that is chronic and inescapable[10] is the most harmful. Stress works directly on the midbrain, triggering the release of cortisol and corticotrophin-releasing factor (CRF), both of which are key neurological ingredients in depression and addiction.[11] As a nonaddict, these neurochemicals and hormones will make you feel anxious and exhausted and make you susceptible to premature aging and a myriad of other diseases. For an addict, in addition to all of that, elevated amounts of these substances in the body sensitize the brain to compulsive and uncontrollable cravings for addictive substances in the following manner.

Stress elevates CRF and cortisol in the blood, the natural "feel okay" dopamine system is repressed, the anhedonic individual encounters a drug, which powerfully (if temporarily) relieves this condition, and the brain interprets this relief as the key to survival itself. We are then off to the races.

In the presence of these chronically elevated stress hormones, and lacking cortical coping mechanisms, the dopamine, or healthy reward, system is suppressed or broken. Stress-related hormones in the blood cause a down regulation, or decrease, in dopamine receptors, and the person becomes anhedonic, unable to experience pleasure in the normally rewarding experiences of life. Although the brain is releasing dopamine in response to these activities, the cells do not receive it. If a person with the genetic burden and elevated levels of cortisol and CRF experiences chronic, unrelievable stress and gets a hold of any addictive substance, the brain is flooded with substances that mirror the effects of dopamine in the brain, and the person finds immediate relief and release. The feeling is, My God, this stuff works! The flood of artificial dopamine is interpreted by the dopamine-starved cells as the most important way of securing one's survival, and securing drugs quickly rises to become the organizing principle of an addict's life.

The fascinating new field of science known as epigenetics (which I'll cover in more detail in chapter 9) also plays a very important role in whether or not we will become addicts. Around fifteen years ago, after the human genome was finally enumerated, many scientists felt that the majority of the job was complete—that we had finally discovered the keys to human life and health. Well, as it turned out, our genetic makeup doesn't tell the whole story. Perhaps even more important than which genetic cards we've been dealt is how our genes turn on or turn off. According to the epigenetic scientists, these mechanisms, both chemical and electromagnetic, control our health, our happiness, our intelligence, our creativity, and so on, to a very large extent—90 percent.[12] This 90 percent is absolutely within the control of our environment. When I say environment, this means our inner as well as our outer environments, or all four quadrants (as we shall explore in the next chapter). And what is the determining factor in how our genes either turn off or turn on? You guessed it, stress.

As I was preparing this chapter for publication, I heard a family physician being interviewed on NPR, who said that fully 60 percent of all the patients he sees are there for stress-related and stress-caused complaints and diseases. Interestingly enough, while enumerating all the diseases that were caused by stress, he did not mention addiction. So not only is stress a major causative factor in the disease of addiction as well as many other life-threatening diseases, but unhealthy stress-coping mechanisms, such as drugs, tobacco, and alcohol, become life-threatening diseases themselves.[13]

According to Dr. Hans Selye,[14] a pioneer in the field of endocrinology who actually coined the term "stress," stress has two poles: di-stress and eu-stress. Distress is the negative stress that we are talking about as a causative factor in many of our diseases, including addiction, and eustress is the positive stress that leads us to create, to grow, and to heal. In our Integral Recovery Practice, we treat for distress and use eustress as a means of transforming our lives and as a clear pathway to sobriety and lifelong health and happiness.

What are the causative factors behind chronic distress and the resulting neurobiological cravings for dopamine? They could be any or all of the following:

1. Chemical imbalance in the brain

2. Unresolved trauma from the past

3. Negative narrative stories about one's self and the world

4. Inability to cope with the present

5. Lack of purpose, meaning, or connection in one's life (also known as existential despair)

6. Toxic relationships. Often these relationships occur between people, but a toxic (stress-inducing, unhealthy) relationship can also be with the place where a person lives, when one is living under a constant threat from which there is no escape, as in a war zone, or an area that has suffered severe environmental degradation.[15]

These causative factors are biological, emotional, cognitive, and spiritual. Without addressing these issues, there is no long-term cure for addiction; by cure I mean reestablishing the locus of control in the neocortex and away from the needy, craving, compulsive, reptilian midbrain.

Addressing these causative factors using the AQAL map as our organizing, three-dimensional framework is what Integral Recovery is all about. This is what will make the difference between long-term sobriety and chronic relapse and death for an addict.

Let's look at these factors individually and see what is to be done.

1. Chemical imbalance in the brain. There is much that can be done in this regard. There are now affordable tests that use saliva and urine to measure the levels of all known essential neurochemicals that factor into the chemical imbalances that cause stress and suffering for the afflicted individual and lead to constant relapse. Prior to this, short of a spinal tap, there was just no way of knowing for sure. A spinal tap is expensive and invasive. This led physicians to look at the symptoms, offer educated guesses, and prescribe medications accordingly. This was a hit-and-miss method at best and led to a lot of tweaking and experimenting with types of medications and dosages. Having been on medications for severe depression, I experienced this dance firsthand. This may also take a long time, which prolongs the suffering and danger to the patient.

    As I used to say to my students, there is simply no dipstick that I can put in your brain and tell you that you are two quarts low on dopamine, one quart low on serotonin, a quart high on cortisol, and about a gallon high on norepinephrine! Well, now the "dipstick" is available. Thank God. We now have affordable procedures that can tell us the levels of all of the essential brain chemicals, and we can track the rebalancing progress, thereby offering our patients and students more effective and efficient treatment. We have a number of ways to do this rebalancing of brain chemistry, which include targeted supplementation, improved diet, medication (if indicated), exercise, and brainwave entrainment meditation.[16] This is excellent news.

2. Unresolved trauma from the past. This is a big one. I have found, more often than not, that in most cases my students have suffered some sort of major trauma in their past.[17] In the late eighties, I befriended a group of homeless men who lived on the streets of San Francisco. Almost all of them were

Vietnam vets who had experienced some real hell during the
war and could not quite make it back into the mainstream of
American life. For the most part, I found them to be great
guys, very loyal to each other, but haunted by demons from
their past. Unresolved trauma also came up frequently among
the young people I worked with for many years in wilderness programs. In the girls' groups, the majority had suffered
some sort of rape or sexual molestation, and this was often
true of the boys groups as well. Remember, just having the
genetic profile is not sufficient in itself; one must also have
an external or internal source of constant, unrelieved stress.
Unreleased trauma is very often the source of this stress. In
another chapter, I will talk about the very specific techniques
I have developed for getting at these repressed materials and
getting free of them.

3. Negative narrative stories about one's self and the world. From
    our lives, histories, and impressions, we all build stories about
    ourselves and the nature of reality. Often, these stories are
    largely unconscious, but they exert tremendous power over
    our lives and brain chemistry. Part of the process of getting
    well in Integral Recovery involves looking at these stories and
    the narratives we have created and seeing how they affect us.
    When they are negative and not optimal, we can see them
    for the creative fictions they are and rewrite them so that
    they are optimal and help us to achieve our goals and create
    the kind of lives that we want to live.

4. Inability to cope with the present. I have found that, almost
    across the board, addicts do not have a healthy ability to cope
    with the day-to-day vagaries of life. Day-to-day events—even
    watching or reading the news—can cause unacceptable levels
    of stress, which lead to a case of the "F___ its!" that is almost
    always a prelude to relapse. One of the most amazing things
    that we have found with brainwave entrainment technology
    is that when you continue to use it on a daily basis, your
    stress threshold continues to rise and that after a number of
    years of dedicated practice, almost nothing can knock you off
    center for long. We become like those punching bag toys we
    had when I was a boy. You slug and whack 'em, and they pop

right back up. With practice, we become resilient and nearly unflappable.

5. Lack of purpose, meaning, or connection in one's life. This is simply not a healthy option for the recovering addict. It has been said that if you have a why you can almost always find a how. Victor Frankl in his classic work, *Man's Search for Meaning,*[18] wrote how his experience in the Nazi death camps taught him that those inmates who found in themselves a reason to live were the ones who survived. As the disease of addiction drags the individual down into toxic egocentric narcissism, the journey of Integral Recovery makes us look for and find what matters to us—what we are willing to live for and to what higher purpose we can dedicate our lives. Viktor Frankl teaches us that happiness is not something that one can successfully pursue as an end in itself, but emerges as a byproduct of our meaningful activities.

6. Toxic relationships. If we understand stress as the ultimate triggering factor of the addictive craving response, it follows that we can treat addiction by reducing stress in the addict's relationships and life circumstances. This involves family therapy, making amends where necessary, and, when needed, leaving behind toxic unhealthy relationships. William Glasser, in his excellent book *Choice Theory,*[19] contends that we have a handful (maybe five or ten) of key relationships in our lives and that how we navigate and negotiate these relationships is a major factor in the quality and happiness that we achieve in our lives. Cleaning up these key relationships, even if the cleaning means ending the relationships in some cases, is one of the ongoing tasks of our Integral Recovery journey.

We must learn to be effective in the world, which means providing for ourselves and those we are responsible for. This includes learning how to work, how to study, how to pay our bills and taxes, and how to meet our responsibilities. It also means learning how to invest, how to be a leader, an entrepreneur, how to actually achieve our dreams and give our gifts to the world. An Integral Recovery model will necessarily include these topics and will provide teachers who have achieved some degree of mastery in these areas.

In addition to becoming successful in our relationships and our work, we must at the same time become successful at navigating our interior worlds, increasing our stress–coping skills, and raising our stress threshold. We must cultivate our interior gardens and grow connections to our strength, wisdom, and love, which will, in turn, bless and illumine all our relations and endeavors. This is precisely what the Integral Recovery model is designed to do.

2

The Integral Map

To break out of prison you need a good map.

—Ken Wilber

The Integral map is also known as the AQAL map. AQAL is an acronym for all quadrants, all lines, all levels, all states, and all types. In the succeeding chapters, we will examine each of these components of the Integral map and see how they apply to the mission of Integral Recovery and how they help us to cover all the essential bases that are necessary for lasting, lifelong recovery.

In Integral Recovery, with the comprehensive outlook provided by the AQAL map's four quadrants, we are able to address our physical health; our inner emotional, spiritual, and intellectual life; our relational life, which includes our relationships to other beings, both human and nonhuman; and our relations with the exterior world, financial, professional, environmental, and technological among others. A simple way to express the four quadrants, which my brilliant wife came up with, is my body, my self, my people, my world. The quadrants allow us to clearly discern the causes and effects of stress in any or all of the quadrants as well as to follow the positive effects of the healing work and practices that we do.

It is important to note that if we can show the physical causes of addiction in the brain, this brings about a major shift in how we view and treat addicts and—equally important—how addicts view and treat themselves. This does not mean that addiction is only found in the Upper-Right (UR), or physical body, quadrant; it simultaneously arises in all other quadrants. That is why we need an all-quadrant approach.

The four quadrants alone might seem like more than enough to give us a very useful and holistic framework in and of themselves; the genius of the AQAL map, however, is that it covers quadrants and much more; the map also includes our developmental stages (or levels) of growth, which we all must come to grips with, both as individuals and as a species. This is particularly important in our quest for recovery because addiction is both progressive and devolutionary, while recovery is progressive and evolutionary. To know and understand the stages we will go through, both during our regression into the disease and our growth through and beyond the disease, is immensely helpful and practical. It provides us with a map of where we are, where we have been, and the possible future that awaits us.

The map includes lines, or intelligences, which show us our strengths, our weaknesses, and what essential capacities have been corrupted by the disease, thus revealing what must be healed and cultivated in a lifelong Integral Recovery Practice. From our lines, we learn not only what has to be worked on, but how to do so and also what an exciting and rewarding process this can be.

From the AQAL map, we also learn to become aware of the basic, everpresent states of consciousness that we experience day to day and moment to moment. We learn what states are and what states aren't and how to negotiate them as they arise. We also learn how these states of consciousness figure into addiction and optimal health. We learn how to use and train states, developing an extraordinary capability that will produce versions of ourselves that we hardly thought possible, as well as leading us to an awareness of what is beyond all states. Ken Wilber has referred to state training as a true "science of happiness."

From the AQAL map's types, we learn to understand and balance the essential polarities of masculine and feminine that we all contain and how we can use this understanding to express and manifest our truest and best selves. In studying types, we also study our personality types and discover how the knowledge of our type and the types of others can lead us to greater understanding and effectiveness in our life.

Sound like a lot? It is. But as we dive into this map of reality, it will be experienced as a great intuitive resonance, a great "Aha!" that will help change, inspire, and heal us. Our wisdom will grow as we practice and live our lives at ever greater depths, with ever more wonder. Ultimately, it will become increasingly clear that this is Work Worth Doing.

Part I of the Map: The Four Quadrants

The four quadrants are four dimensions of reality that are present on every occasion and cannot be effectively reduced to one another. AQAL did not invent these dimensions; they have always been there. They are lenses on reality, through which we look at the interiors and exteriors of individuals and collectives. Being aware of these aspects of reality is tremendously useful in providing us with skillful means with which to approach recovery.

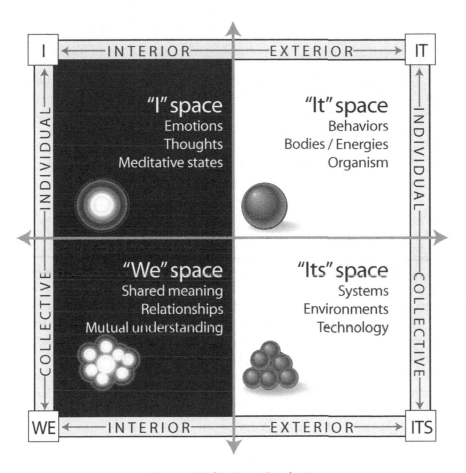

Figure 1. The Four Quadrants

The UR quadrant represents the exterior of the individual. By exterior, I mean the physical body: the organs, circulatory system, muscles, brain chemistry, bones, and so forth. This is the traditional territory of Western medicine. It is physical; it can be touched, measured, weighed, dissected, and analyzed chemically. The fundamental perspective of the UR quadrant is that of "it." This is the individual objective dimension.

The Upper–Left (UL) quadrant represents the interiors of the individual: thoughts, feelings, emotions, and beliefs. The perspective of this quadrant is that of "I." It is the individual subjective dimension. Our interiors are very real and present, but you could not take your love for your family, weigh it, put it in a box, and hand it back to me. Your love is not a physical object. We could try and identify your love by taking a snapshot of your brain using an EEG or other device that would show us what part of your brain was firing when you experienced feelings of love, but in the end it would tell us nothing about what experiencing your feelings is like for you. You have to tell us about your experience for us to understand you. We can then compare it to our own and others' similar experiences and begin to have a better understanding of your interior reality.

The Lower–Left (LL) quadrant is the "we" space, or plural interiors, the collective subjective dimension. Our individual interiors are happening all the time, but when we communicate, we create a "we" space, a field of mutual understanding. Again, this is an interior in that it has no locality. We can't see a shared understanding or cultural belief, even though it is very real.

Last, we have the Lower–Right (LR) quadrant. This represents our plural exteriors, and the perspective is that of "its." It is the collective objective dimension, which includes all the "out there" world: nature, the internet, highways, the economy, the whole magnificent web of life.

In an Integral approach, we say that all of these dimensions or quadrants must be included. Why? Because in Integral Recovery we define health as a healthy balance in all four quadrants. The reverse holds equally true. The disease of addiction is a disease of all four quadrants: in the UR quadrant, it is a brain disease; in the UL quadrant, it is an interior spiritual and emotional disease; in the LL quadrant, it is a relational disease; and in the LR quadrant, it is a social disease that attacks the fabric of our civilization and drains our treasure as well as the gifts and contributions of millions of people.

It turns out that most human endeavors, including the treatment of addiction, tend to unconsciously favor certain quadrants over others. In traditional recovery, treatment often focuses only on the inner life—past traumas, emotional imbalances, and so on—and neglects to consider physical health or brain chemistry. Or conversely, a doctor might treat only the physical you, without taking the trouble to consider your emotional and mental states. Instead of an either/or approach, Integral Recovery is a yes/and approach—both interior and exterior, individual and collective.

A further insight the quadrants give us is that any gains made in any of the quadrants will help stabilize and lift up the others. Likewise, any stressors in any of the quadrants will place a burden on all other quadrants. The four quadrants allow us to make a comprehensive diagnostic map of the damage done in each area, which then points the way to the steps that need to be taken to maintain sobriety, restore balance in each quadrant, and grow toward optimal health.

For example, if you are a couch potato subsisting on a diet of beer and fast food, your UR quadrant (physical health) will, in short order, be devastated. (See the film *Super-Size Me*.) This will, in turn, affect your moods, your relations with your family, and possibly your job and finances. If, on the other hand, you detoxify your body, start eating nutritionally life-enhancing foods, and begin a program of rigorous exercise, we will rightly expect to see remarkable improvements in your bodily health and vigor. At the same time, we will see improvements in your moods and outlook (UL quadrant), as well as in your relations with family, friends, and the outside world in terms of employment, effectiveness, and the ability to do what is necessary to support health and happiness (LL and LR quadrants).

In the Integral model, we work on all four dimensions simultaneously: we build a strong body, we clean up and expand our interiors, we heal our relations to others, and we pay our bills, provide for our families, heal our environment, and make sure that the oil gets changed. When a client enters Integral treatment, one of the first steps is to perform a four-quadrant assessment of their life situation.

Not only do the four quadrants help us evaluate a client's situation, but I teach it to my clients as a part of their recovery practice to help them begin to make sense of their life as well. As we learn and apply the AQAL map, looking at phenomena this way becomes second nature. And if we have data missing from any of the four quadrants, then we know automatically that we are dealing with an incomplete picture.

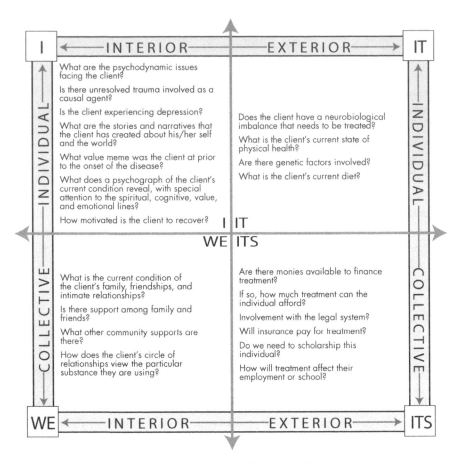

Figure 2. Four-Quadrant Treatment Assessment

Let's take a hypothetical but very common situation. Let's say we have a student that has been on a methamphetamine binge for six months. There are going to be huge and obvious issues in the UR quadrant. Our student's brain chemistry will be out of balance and severely depleted of essential neurotransmitters such as serotonin and dopamine. It is likely he will also be nutritionally depleted from taking the drug and eating very little. There may be sores on his body, which are becoming infected from picking at his skin (a behavior often associated with methamphetamine use). Often we find that methamphetamine addicts are very promiscuous in their sexual practices, which of course leads to a myriad of sexually transmitted diseases, including HIV.

In the UL quadrant, our student will be experiencing fear, anger, cravings, depression, despair, in short, an emotional roller coaster ride. In the LL quadrant, his relationships with family, friends, and colleagues will likely be in shambles due to lying and stealing, and, finally, psychotic behaviors brought about by extended use of methamphetamines. In the LR quadrant, there will probably be a myriad of issues and damages brought about by the acting out associated with methamphetamine use. Our student will, more than likely, be broke, his health insurance may have lapsed, and there may be outstanding warrants, bad debts, and so forth.

While we identify the genesis of addiction as starting in the UR quadrant because it is a brain disease, we have also shown how the disease of addiction causes catastrophe in all three other quadrants. Recently, in our Integral Recovery (IR) treatment program, we have increased the focus on the LR quadrant and added a LR coach to our staff as, oftentimes, by the time a student reaches us for treatment their LR quadrant is a complete disaster: they have failed to pay bills, tickets, credit cards, health insurance, and mortgages, and there are all sorts of mounting debts and other life stressors that seem absolutely overwhelming from the perspective of early recovery. All of this can lead to despair, stress, and shame, as in, "I will never be able to make this right, so what's the point?" The increase in stress, as we have shown before, can lead to relapse as well as other financial and legal issues.

The LR coach takes the time to identify what issues can and need to be dealt with for each student. Then, one thing at a time, issue by issue, step by step, the bills get paid, the phone calls get made—restitutions have begun. While this may take a while (Rome was not destroyed in a day and will not be rebuilt in a day) we have found that each time a step is taken or an issue is resolved, there is a new sense of hope and empowerment: I can actually deal with this. Among our students, we've seen a new desire emerge, to take responsibility for one's life situations and get that which was formerly chaotic back under control.

Another improvisation we have recently instituted at Integral Recovery is a workshop called Getting Things Done.[2] Here students are trained in how to organize and prioritize their lives and responsibilities. Again, we have found this to be very inspiring as students begin to learn how to actually get things done: once a need is defined and put on a context-appropriate list, it can then be transformed from a nagging, gotta-get-this-done chore to an objectified, achievable task. By the way, this practice is also very helpful for our staff and yours truly.

Each one of these steps and accomplishments in the LR quadrant leads to more life integration, functionality, and coherence—which is another way of saying Integral Recovery. An organized and functional LR approach to life and its challenges creates a firm and highly functional foundation for our dreams, visions, and aspirations, which otherwise often become neglected and given up on under the weight of mounting financial, legal, and other LR issues.

Beyond the typical profile of a methamphetamine addict, we might find the following (di)stresses caused in all four quadrants by the disease of addiction:

- Upper-Right quadrant: health problems such as heart disease, emphysema, cancer, HIV and other sexually transmitted diseases, pneumonia, malnutrition, and damage caused to the body by the violence that often accompanies a drug-centered life.

- Upper-Left quadrant: anger, despair, cravings, depression, psychosis.

- Lower-Left quadrant: neglected children, neglected family, broken homes, divorces, family violence, gang violence, criminal associations, less than harmonious relations with law enforcement, etc.

- Lower-Right quadrant: legal charges and convictions, ever-accumulating debt, neglect and abuse of the environment (such as when meth lab operators pour their toxic chemical byproducts into our land and water), homelessness, health insurance lapse, and chronic poverty in our inner cities and elsewhere, such as the devastation that is found on many Native American reservations.

Given this understanding of addiction that the four quadrants enable us to see, an Integral treatment program would necessarily address the issues present in all four quadrants. Here's what a four-quadrant Integral treatment plan would look like:

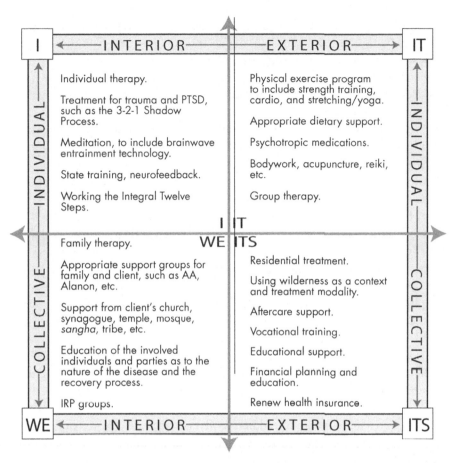

Figure 3. Four-Quadrant Treatment Plan

Starting with the UR quadrant, the physical effects of addiction must be addressed. This includes damage to the functioning of the brain and other organs. Treatment modalities necessary to address the above issues are nutrition and the establishment of a healthy diet, that is, organic and nonchemical-laden, supplementation, brainwave entrainment technology, cranial electrical stimulation, and exercise (strength training, cardio, and yoga).

Treatment for causes and effects of stress in the UL quadrant would include meditation, contemplative prayer, individual therapy, trauma and shadow work, and the use of affirmations and visualizations.

Focusing on the LL quadrant, treatment could include couples therapy, family therapy, the building of an Integral practice-friendly culture and support group, other support groups such as AA or NA, religious affiliations with churches, temples, mosques, whichever is appropriate, and restorative work to heal the damages done to relationships due to drug-compelled activities.

To treat issues in the LR quadrant, we find or create supportive, healthy living environments, cleaning out toxic elements from our living environments, reestablish our relationship with nature, take care of the business of living, house payments, car payments, bank accounts, educational needs, and financial planning, to name but some.

Healing and restoration will not happen overnight, and the first part of the journey is simply to get well. I often tell my students that it took quite a while to make such an absolute mess of their life and it's going to take a bit of time to sort it all out and make things right. What we don't want to do is try to "fix" things before we are ready. This will simply lead to more failure, stress, and relapse. "First things first" is one of the classic bits of wisdom from AA that we want to bring along on our Integral Recovery journey.

By using the four quadrants, we can identify the major effects of addiction that need to be accounted for and treated as well as the causes of stress that will keep the individual addicted, unhappy, and unhealthy. If we neglect any of these causative and primary sources of stress, our patients and clients who are addicts will not get well. (And you'll never get back the money they owe you.) The four quadrants are an essential tool and are truly the doorway to Integral health and consciousness, where everything that matters is included, not neglected.

3

Stages and Spiral Dynamics

"Every age but ours, had its model, its ideal . . . About all we have left is a well-adjusted man without problems, a very pale and doubtful substitute. Perhaps we shall soon be able to use as our guide and model the fully growing and self-fulfilling human being, the one in whom his potentialities are coming to full development, the one whose inner nature expresses itself freely, rather than being warped, repressed, or denied."

—Abraham Maslow, *Toward a Psychology of Being*, 1962

Introduction to Stages

One of the ways that the AQAL map brings radical new depth to the field of recovery is with the inclusion of developmental stages. Adding developmental knowledge and dimension gives us a directional compass in the quest for Integral Recovery. It allows us to understand that our current developmental altitude is not the ultimate view—it is just where we presently find ourselves. This understanding engenders healthy humility as well as inspiration for the journey ahead. As one spiritual master put it, "It is good to know what's above you." Stages offer us a revolutionary way of comprehending ourselves and our world and help us to make a great leap forward in our understanding of addiction and its progression. I often tell my students that if they understand stages, they will never look at the world in the same old way. This is a great lead in, and I have never had anyone dispute this claim after grasping the system. There is frequently a wonder that borders on a sense of revelation as they begin to understand their own struggles, family dynamics, and the conflicts and possibilities in the world around them.

In Integral theory, stages are levels of consciousness, stable and lasting like rungs on a ladder. They determine changes in altitude, which, once attained, are always available. A stage of development can be likened to the acquisition of language. Once you have it, you don't lose it (in the absence of catastrophic brain trauma). You don't wake up in the morning and think, "Whoops! I forgot how to talk." Or imagine it this way: You are building a structure and you complete the fourth floor. The floor has been built—it is not going to disappear at midnight, turn into a pumpkin, or go away when it rains. Although the inhabitants of the house may not always be on the fourth floor, they always have access to it. Each floor represents a stage of consciousness.

When I wake up in the morning, before tea, coffee, or meditation, I may not be on my highest psychic floor yet (most likely not), but I can make my way there. One of the most fascinating things about stages is that with deep meditation and our Integral Recovery Practice (IRP), we not only have access to our current stage of development, but we can go back to our earlier stages and clean out the trash in the basement that could be causing us a lot of trouble. We also have occasional glimpses of our potential future growth, which is inspiring and lightens our load as we continue the climb to become our best and highest selves.

Achieving new stages is generally hard work—especially if you are pushing into stages above the dominant level, or center of gravity, of your family, your peer group, or your culture. In this case, the dominant center of gravity will pull you down and make upward growth difficult and challenging, requiring concerted and even heroic effort to scale these heights. At the same time, if you are at a stage of development below the cultural norm, gravity will pull you up and facilitate your progress up the ladder, up the spiral, as the norms and structures are firmly in place to support this level of development.

For Integral Recovery treatment providers, identifying a client's developmental level enables them to function with much greater skill in dealing with the client's needs and in developing an individualized IRP. Treatment providers are able to speak to their clients "where they're at," in ways that clients understand and resonate with, allowing for far more effective communication and hence treatment.

There are many stage models of development we could use in Integral Recovery, but for our purposes Spiral Dynamics is, I believe, the most useful and compelling model. Spiral Dynamics not only maps our developmental values from birth to whatever high and lofty levels we might obtain, but also maps our moral development as a species, thereby offering us rich new insights into the cultural landscape of the human family. But before we look at Spiral Dynamics in detail, let's look at psychological development from an even more basic starting point, which will give us a solid foundation for that which is to follow.

Egocentric, Ethnocentric, Worldcentric, and Kosmocentric

The first level we talk about is the egocentric level. What do you care about at this level? I, me, mine. This is an early, primitive stage of moral development and, as we shall see, is where most addicts end up in the latter progression of the disease of addiction no matter where they were at the outset. A formerly caring family member or responsible citizen quickly arrives at a very unhealthy, egocentric altitude where the attitude is, "Screw you! Nothing matters but me and staying high." At this level of the disease, other people become objects to be opposed or manipulated in order to secure a supply of the addictive substance(s).

The next level up is ethnocentric. At the ethnocentric level, you care not only about yourself, but also about your family, tribe, nation, team, however you draw the circle of inclusion. Based on many years of experience, I believe that this is the first level where effective recovery can begin. There are very good and logical arguments for egocentric recovery (i.e., "You will die if you keep using!"), but that level's defiance, lack of humility, and "Don't you dare tell me what to do" attitude make the work of recovery (which requires listening to others and doing what they tell you) very difficult and nearly impossible. I have personally never seen it work very well.

Quickly into the process of recovery, you must come to the realization that this disease is *not* just about yourself, but directly and adversely affects those closest to you. The denial structure of the disease, when the reptilian brain is running the show, often makes this realization seem like a revelation in early recovery, and it brings about very healthy, stage-appropriate feelings of guilt. As the fog of denial begins to lift, the reality and the consequences of your crimes, betrayals, and addictive behaviors become increasingly and painfully clear. The task then becomes not just to clean yourself up, but to clean up the messes you have made (in all four quadrants) and the unjustified hurt and suffering that you have visited on others, often upon those about whom you care the most.

Following ethnocentric, the next rung is worldcentric. At this level, you are able to consider your program of recovery and your commitment

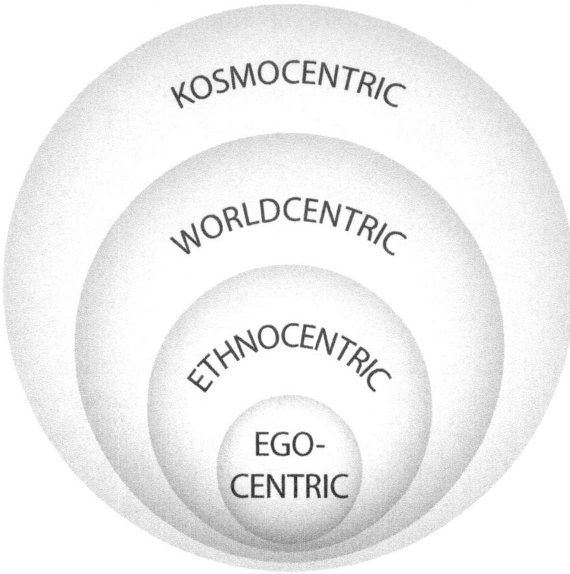

Figure 4. Levels/Stages of Moral Development[1]

to it from a much larger perspective—one that includes what is good for you and your people (however they are defined), as well as how your choices affect everyone. The win, win of ethnocentric becomes the win, win, win of worldcentric.

The highest level on this simplified scale is kosmocentric. In the Integral model, we use the "k" to connote the Greek Pythagorean sense of the cosmos, which includes consciousness, art, creativity, and so on as essential elements of the universe along with the material universe. At the kosmocentric level, the person includes the entire universe (beyond the human) in her consideration and care. Integral developmental psychologist Susanne Cook-Greuter[2] describes this level as unitive, or "unitive consciousness," where we have moved beyond our strictly individual ego-, ethnic-, or even world-identification to an identification with all life and all beings, past, present, and future. This is not merely an intellectual, cognitive realization, but also a full-bodied, lived experience.

One very interesting thing about this developmental map is that while most people who show up for treatment in the latter stages of addiction have their center of gravity at an egocentric level, with the help of Integral treatment, students are able to shift their center of gravity quite rapidly back to the level they held prior to the addiction gaining control over their life. Those who began their addictive journey into hell at an egocentric level should also be able to progress quickly to an ethnocentric level, due to the transformative and evolutionary power of IRP.

As Ken Wilber notes in his opus magnum, *Sex, Ecology, Spirituality*, deep interior work is actually an anecdote for narcissism.[3] As we continue to go inside and tap into our essence, deconstructing our conditioning and our unconscious knots, the hold of the narcissistic trance begins to lose its power to control us, and, I might add, the same is true of the addictive trance. So, meditation, far from being a self-absorbed, narcissistic act, of which it has sometimes been accused, is actually a way out of narcissism and our own self-absorption, because as we deepen our emotional and spiritual work, we become more connected to the world and are able to offer our services in a skillful and compassionate way.

It is important to note that each higher level includes the cares and concerns of the prior levels, while at the same time transcending those levels. For example, at the ethnocentric level, you still don't want to be thrown out of your house, but at this point you also care about your family. I would say that at each higher level, the responsibility taken will stick longer, and the choices made will be more powerful—basically because there is more to care about. At the deepest levels, it is the love that we hold for ourselves and others that will be the most powerful motivator to stick with our practices and become our optimal selves.

Now that we have established the basic evolutionary trajectory that moves from primitive values, which only include self or ego, to ethnocentric, worldcentric, and kosmocentric, let us look at Dr. Clare Graves' brilliant model[4] for the new eyes and clarity it can bring to our task of implementing a truly Integral approach to recovery from addiction.

Spiral Dynamics

The story goes that, in the 1950s, Clare Graves was a professor at Union College in Schenectady, New York, teaching introductory psychology to his students. After Graves presented each popular school of psychology (Freudian, Jungian, behaviorist, humanistic, etc.), his students would ask, "Which one is the right one?" Spiral Dynamics[5] was born out of Graves' struggle to make sense of the apparently contradictory theories and answer the question. His answer was that each school of thought was correct on the level that it dealt with.

For example, Freudian psychology tends to deal with early childhood development; in fact, Freudians seem to think that most of our future is determined by what happens in our early relationships with our mothers and fathers and during toilet training. Jungian psychology, however, deals with a completely different area of psychic development, principally archetypes and spiritual "individuation." Behavioral psychology deals with exteriors, or right-hand quadrants, while virtually denying the existence of the Upper-Left quadrant. Finally, humanistic psychology seems to work best with those who have already achieved some level of ego development and maturity. So the story goes that as Graves began to look at this data, an understanding of developmental levels emerged, which then went on to become what we call Spiral Dynamics.

Spiral Dynamics has been tested on over fifty thousand subjects in first, second, and third world countries, and has been found to work cross-culturally in all of these diverse environments. As we began to explore above, Spiral Dynamics offers a hugely important and effective lens to look at human development, both individual and collective. Not only does it help us understand where we are at, but also where we have been and where we are going. Spiral Dynamics helps us understand ethical and moral development as an existential response to ever-changing environmental conditions (in all four quadrants).

As we examine Spiral Dynamics more closely, I believe it will soon become abundantly clear how this tool can add greater understanding and effectiveness to any situation involving our species and how it is an extraordinary tool in understanding and treating addiction. By adding this vertical developmental understanding to treatment, we go a very long way in addressing some of the major issues that have, in the past, stood in the way of developing effective, attractive, and responsive treatment methods.

Let's take a basic overview and see how Spiral Dynamics illuminates the landscape we must inhabit and traverse in our journey of Integral Recovery. Developmental stages in Spiral Dynamics are color coded, and unfold sequentially. They describe eight levels of world views (called "value memes") that human beings can evolve through over the course of a lifetime. This is an open-ended system that allows for a lot of variation at each particular level, and no discernible upper limit to evolution and growth. Everyone is born at square one and moves on from there. The *to be continued...*

Unitive Self
Witness Self. Action and non-action without attachment to outcome.
Realization as a verb not a destination. Apex Self.
Quest: Realizing integrated, free functioning human being.

Holistic Self
Collective Individualism - starting 30 years ago.
Authentic irony. An ecology of perspectives.
Quest: Peace in an incomprehensible world.
AQAL spirituality. Transrational perceptions.
Aware of AQAL arising. Pitfalls: Pathologies of the soul.

Integral Self
World-Kosmocentric - starting 50 years ago.
Healthy hierarchies. Live fully and responsibly.
Integrate the whole spiral. **Quest**: Integral synthesis
to balance the whole with holarchy.
Evolutionary streams awaken, integrate diversity with
discernment, developmental perspective.
Pitfalls: Aborted self-actualization, existential angst...

. . . a radical leap in being . . .

Sensitive Self Age 15–21 yrs. Social Democracies, informational - starting
150 years ago. Pluralism. Seek peace within a caring community. Power with,
solidarity, human rights. **Quest**: Peace, affectionate relations, dialogue and
consensus. **Method**: Appreciate diversity, listen well, consensus.
Pitfalls: Nihilism, inauthenticity, excessive relativism, endless consensus.

Rational Self Age 9–14 yrs. Capitalistic Democracies - starting 300 yrs ago.
Scientific rationalism, worldcentric. Act from self-interest by playing the
game to win. Market-driven meritocracy. **Quest**: Rational truth, material
pleasure, in defense of civilization. **Method**: Science, learn to excel, set goals,
achieve, stats. **Pitfalls**: Scientism, flatland, identity crisis, role confusions,
consumerism, ecological crisis, workaholism, goal-fixation, denial of spirit.

Rule/Role Self Age 7-8 yrs. Late Mythic, Nation States, Authoritarian,
Absolutistic Religious - starting 5,000 yrs ago. Ethnocentric, life has meaning,
direction, and purpose. **Quest**: Ultimate peace, good vs evil. **Method**: Fit in,
follow the given rules, discipline, faith. **Pitfalls**: fundamentalism, fascism, etc.

Power Self Age 3–6 yrs. Early Mythic, Feudal & Exploitive Empire -10,000 yrs.
Aggression, might makes right, be and do what you want. **Quest**: Heroic status,
power, glory, and revenge. **Method**: Align with power, take what you need,
power over others, force. **Pitfalls**: Gangs, anxiety, phobias, bullying, terrorism.

Magic/Animistic Self Age 1-3 yrs . Tribal Order - starting 50,000 yrs ago.
Egocentric, impulsive. Keep the spirits happy and tribe's nest warm and safe.
Magical thinking. **Quest**: Safe mode of living, security. **Method**: Petition to
Gods with ritual. **Pitfalls**: Borderline, narcissism, omnipotentcy, tribal conflicts.

Instinctive Self Age 0-18 months. Survival Bands - starting 100,000 yrs ago.
Do what you must to stay alive. Un-differentiated, narcissism.
Quest: Food, water, warmth, shelter. **Methods**: Scavenge whatever you need.
Pitfalls: Primitive developmental psycho-pathologies, autism.

Figure 5. Integral Spiral of Development[6]

unfolding stages not only track our individual progress up the spiral, but also our evolutionary emergence as a species. What keeps the spiral active and evolving is that the solutions for the challenges at each emergent level can only be answered and met at the next higher stage, which in turn has its own conflicts that are only resolved at the next higher stage, and so on. Thus, the problems and issues of an addict, whom the disease of addiction has dragged down to an unhealthy and toxic egocentric level, can only be resolved and addressed as a healthy ethnocentric level comes online (or back online, as the case may be).[7]

The color *beige—Instinctive Self*—represents the first stage. This is where we are all born; our ancestors inhabited this domain one hundred thousand years ago plus. The ethical concerns at this level are simple sensory motor survival issues. This is the terrain in the first eighteen months of life in a normal developmental process. Our ancestors at this point were living in small bands, and their main concern was eating and not being eaten.

The next stage emerged around fifty thousand years ago and is called *purple—Magic Animistic Self*. Purple represents the shamanistic, magical, animistic stage of human development, represented beautifully in the Lascaux cave paintings in Southern France. At this stage, the world is full of spirits that must be propitiated and communicated with through rituals and sacrifice. The end value espoused here is safety in a powerful, often frightening world of nature dominated by mysterious forces.

In normal development, we pass through this wave at one to three years old. Here, a child lives in a magical world, where, if he pulls the covers over his head, he can't be seen because he cannot see you. The clouds in the sky follow him as he walks. Pretty primitive stuff this, but it was at the leading edge of evolution fifty thousand years ago. As the purple stage emerged, our ancestors were able to organize themselves into larger tribal structures that centered around blood and kinship; human sacrifice was often the order of the day.

The next level that came about (and this is where it starts getting interesting for our purposes) was *red—Impulsive Self*. Red kicked in as a major force around ten thousand years ago. This is the egocentric power level and is represented in the Greco-Roman gods, the Nordic gods, the Meso-American gods, and so on. At this point in our development, there was no sense of an all-powerful, all-wise deity. The gods were like super heroes with generally bad attitudes. They were mean, lustful, jealous, and seemed to derive pleasure out of messing with humans. In short, they can be seen as personifications and projections of the red selfish and impulsive ego structure.[8]

In our culture, you see this level of development negatively represented in prison gangs and street gangs. Reds are narcissistic, selfish, impulsive, and basically amoral. Reds are capable of taking only one perspective: their own. This is an important level to understand, as, in my experience, when the disease of addiction takes over and progresses, the moral level of the addict devolves or slides back down the spiral to an unhealthy, egocentric red—no matter what stage the addict had attained prior to the onset of the disease. This is shocking to watch from the outside, if it is happening to someone you know and love. It is the horrifying transformation of a person from their Dr. Jekyll healthy self into the psychopathic Mr. Hyde.

This is not hyperbole. It is the transformation that occurs in addiction: we become walking, craving, lying, impulsive, manipulative creatures controlled by the overpowering wants of our primitive, reptilian brains. Addiction is progressive in that the disease advances along predictable lines but *regressive* in that no matter what level was attained prior to the addiction's onset, the addict will end up at a pathological red, egocentric stage or lower, with occasional flashes of the old pre-addict self shining through. Others are no longer "thou" in the sense that Martin Buber spoke of, but "it," merely objects to be manipulated, lied to, stolen from, or eliminated, if they threaten the supply of the addictive substance in any way. There is a joke that I often tell in classes with addicts or their families. It goes like this. "How do you know when an addict is lying?" Answer: "When his lips are moving." This does not produce shame in addicts as one might think but is most often met with nervous laughter and relief, as in, "Somebody understands what we've been going through."

As the reptilian brain and its cravings take over a person's life, all the higher emotional and intellectual capacities are subjugated to the totalitarian dictatorship of a sick and craving brain. This cancels out about five thousand years of human moral development. If the addict survives long enough, unchecked, this regression can take them all the way down to beige. Imagine the addict or alcoholic living in a cardboard box in a back alley, or under a bridge, who emerges only for brief forays to get more drugs and maybe a little food: one hundred thousand years of human development down the drain of addiction.

Traditionally, in our society, it has been organized sports and the military that have served as rites of passage to get young red-meme men to blue. The training goes something like this: You are less than nothing and here's a big surprise for you. You are not the center of the universe. You are going to learn to obey the rules. You are going to learn to work together. You are going to learn discipline, and you are going to earn the right to be part of this team . . . a soldier, football player, marine, and so on. Sound familiar? I was in the army, and I was amazed to watch a bunch of shucking and jiving young men turn into tough, disciplined soldiers in short order under the artful and often brilliant care of our drill sergeants.

This is an important point because in the early phase of treatment we often deal with people at a very sick red level of development. This means that the treatment providers, while being compassionate (which literally means "to suffer with"), need to speak to clients at the level they are currently at. In red's case, this means being firm and direct and calling a spade a spade (which would not work with a green-meme person—whom you'll meet later). In early treatment things need to be very structured and directive; this is the program, we get up at such and such a time, do yoga, meditate, start class at 10:00 . . . hit the gym at 3:00, and so on. There is not a lot of wiggle room and down time, except to work on assignments and possibly catch up on sleep. Structure, discipline, honesty, and consequences are all things that reds might not like but can respect and understand. This is why recovering addicts and alcoholics are often very good teachers, because they know all the cons and self-deceptions that addicts are prone to, and addicts in early recovery know that they know.

From red we move to *blue—Rule—Role Self*. Blue began to emerge about five thousand years ago. This is the stage of absolutist, fundamentalist religion. It first began in the era historians call "the Axial Age," as in an axle, or age of a great turning. This is when the leaders and prophets of the great wisdom traditions were first teaching and transforming their worlds. This age basically started with the Vedic sages of ancient India and went on to include the likes of Buddha, Lao Tzu, Jesus, Zoroaster, and Plato, and probably ended with Muhammad. All founders of the great religions in this period taught some version of greater kindness, forgiveness, and the Golden Rule. This was the great "turning." Turning from what? Turning from the bloody and cruel excesses of red-dominated civilizations.

Remember, all vertical stage growth happens in response to environmental pressures and problems that the current stage does not address sufficiently or successfully. Blue brought in the healing balm of a Higher Power that was good, as opposed to jealous and capricious. The concept arose of a holy or divinely chosen community, based on purpose, ultimate peace, sacred writings and teachings, hierarchy, and humility, where ego desires become subservient to a Higher Authority. This was a huge moral leap from the cruel and often chaotic compulsions of red, reflected again in the egocentric, amoral chaos of late-stage addiction.

In most cases, AA provides a healthy blue structure for newly recovering addicts: go to meetings, get a sponsor, work the steps, and do what God and your sponsor tell you to. This is dead-on correct in that structure, discipline, and accountability are exactly what are needed for many early recovering addicts and alcoholics to experience red-to-blue growth. It only becomes a problem when recovery to blue is actually *not* the end goal of the process—when one is aiming for higher-level development or trying to regain the level or altitude the addict had attained prior to the onset of the disease. Early recovery often needs to be a healthy blue-like structure, but Integral Recovery must help and facilitate recovery to the healthiest prior-inhabited level of development, and higher, if this is feasible and desired by the recovering addict.

Again, the gifts of blue are humility, service to a higher good, and respect for higher authority—all of which are antidotes for the problems created by red: rebellion for rebellion's sake, self-centeredness, and impulsivity. These traits make recovery very doubtful at the red stage, because one definition of an addict is one who can't stop the downward spiral of using without outside help, and a red "Screw you, don't tell me what to do!" attitude makes it very difficult. This is where law enforcement and the court system can be of great assistance in getting addicts into treatment, because our red addicts do understand power and threats to their autonomy. The Damoclean sword of jail time dangling over one's head can be a fantastic initial motivator, but eventually the motivation toward health and recovery must come from within and from a higher altitude than red has at its disposal. So, how do we facilitate growth from red to blue? By speaking to red and framing the practice in language that red can understand. This basic technique applies to change at any level of the spiral.

Blue is a great moral leap forward from the bloody chaos of red, but definitely brings its own set of problems that can then only be resolved at the next stage of development, orange. Blue moves us from egocentric first person (me) to ethnocentric second person (we), where one cares not just about oneself but for the group (family, tribe, nation, religious community, AA group, however one draws that circle). The problem with blue is that it only allows for one perspective or accepted Truth, and anyone outside of that circle of inclusion or care is the "other," in many cases seen as the enemy to be enslaved, converted, or eliminated. As Ken Wilber is fond of saying, "The Nazis loved their children."

The next stage to emerge in our history and on our personal journey is the *orange—Achiever Self.* Some scholars say that one of the major catalysts of the emergence of orange was the "Black Death," which swept through Europe in the late 1340s and killed from one-third to two-thirds of the entire population of Europe. At this point, it was clear to many that the priests, the relics, and the pope—the whole basic mythic structure—were useless in confronting this horrible plague. In fact, the superstitious belief that cats were the consorts of witches and needed, therefore, to be killed led to an increase of the rat population, who carried the fleas that spread the disease. The attitude that began to take root was, to quote Sgt. Friday, "Just the facts, ma'am."[9] The old answers were no longer meeting current challenges and conditions.

Orange began to show up most strongly, at least in the West, around three hundred years ago. The profound flowering of orange came with the advent of the American Revolution, the U.S. Constitution, and the Bill of Rights. Orange was characterized by a progressive moving away from the mythic, medieval blue meme into a much more rational, scientific world view. With orange emerged the scientific method, or rationalism, individualism, modern democracy, the Industrial Revolution, and capitalism. Orange brought us the technological revolution that has swept the world and is continuing to transform our lives as the power of our technology increases exponentially. On an individual level, the person at an orange center of gravity values success, individual freedom, achievement, technology, and skillfulness. The idea is that life is a game; there are winners and losers; the winners get the rewards and the losers don't.

One of the important shifts that occurs when orange emerges is the ability to take multiple perspectives. Orange can move from a second-person, ethnocentric perspective to a third-person, multiple perspective, or worldcentric perspective. Good examples of this are the Declaration of Independence, the United States Constitution, the outlawing of slavery, and the Universal Rights of Man (the rights of women to vote came through orange; women's liberation would continue into green and beyond as the shift from orange to green began to shake the foundations of our society with the emergence of the counterculture in the sixties).

The manifold creativity and inventiveness of orange (or modernity) can be seen everywhere, and a list of orange's incredible accomplishments would be too long to cite here. But along with orange's amazing fecundity came orange's dark and negative aspects, as with all stages on the spiral. Orange's negative aspects can be seen in the runaway greed of unregulated capitalism, the overemphasis on individual rights to the detriment of the common good, and the push for short-term profit over the long-term health of the commons, be it the health of humans or our natural environment. For all of its problems, orange has given us many, many gifts, and we shall need these gifts in abundance in our quest for Integral recovery.

So how does an orange level of development relate to addiction? When you're dealing with an orange in recovery, you can really start talking science: brain chemistry, brainwave entrainment, brainwave states, epigenetics, and so forth. As ever more scientific data becomes available, helping us to better understand the disease of addiction, recovery takes on a whole new dimension and the number of scientifically based practices that can be included in an IRP just keeps on growing.

Enter *green—Sensitive Self*. Green began emerging as a powerful force in the United States around fifty years ago.[10] Among Green's many contributions are the civil rights movement, the environmental movement, women's rights, gay rights, animal rights, and rights for just about any marginalized group that was seen as neglected and misused by the dominant orange center of gravity. Green was a reaction against the often cutthroat, laissez-faire practices of orange and unhealthy capitalism. Green represents an extremely high level of moral development and stands squarely against the marginalization of any group or minority (except for largely rejecting orange and blue). Green rejects classism, racism, sexism, and discrimination of any kind. Everyone is invited to the party; everyone deserves respect and even nurturing. Much goodness has come out of green.

Certainly, new issues and problems have also arisen with the emergence of green. Green attempts to level all values and perspectives to equal status, for to do otherwise would be oppressive, hierarchical, and judgmental. However, all-inclusive, nonjudgmental compassion can mean that green has trouble making judgments at all, since all truth claims are of equal value. Not that there isn't great value in many of green's critiques of past and present injustices, as in Voltaire's rallying cry for the French Revolution, "Remember the cruelties!" However, on the downside, when no truth claim is any more valid than another, the only truth is that there is no truth that is truer than any other truth, at least no absolute truth, which is accepted absolutely! This is a performative contradiction, in which the truth claim contradicts itself, and can quickly become a moral, intellectual, and spiritual dead end. A successful green meeting often consists of everyone getting a chance to share their feelings, since opinions, especially strong ones, are suspect and possibly oppressive. Peaceful communion is the goal. This green moral high ground can often turn into an irresolute swamp, however, where nothing actually gets done.

The traps and pitfalls on the journey to higher consciousness are many. For those at green, the sirens' song of nihilistic, narcissistic relativism can sink the ship and end the journey. You have your truth; I have mine; it's all the same. But ultimately, green's compassion and desire to help heal the world provide a safe harbor so that the journey can continue.

Above the green stage, Graves found something very remarkable indeed. Instead of the next stage or rung in the ladder, he discovered a whole new tier, second tier. Remember, at first tier, all the stages think their perspective is the only right one, whether it is an ethnocentric blue perspective or a kosmocentric green perspective. At second tier, however, the realization emerges that each preceding stage is part of the great evolutionary unfolding of our species, and each one is a component part of the spiral; each stage is needed, and each has its gifts and its part to play to fulfill the symphony of life. The second-tier approach is to adopt a pastoral attitude toward the entire spiral, working to help each level express itself in its healthiest manifestation. At second tier, we become accepting of all the stages rather than rejecting that which came before. Again, we all start at beige. There was never a person born at green or orange. The task becomes to assist everyone to be the best possible versions of themselves and bring forth that which is good and appropriate at each stage, since we need the gifts that each stage brings.

First Tier

Before we continue our brief survey of the human developmental spiral, let's look at where we have been and where we are going. Clare Graves called the first six stages we have looked at the *first tier*. Before we look at the next emerging stage, let's examine the characteristics shared by all the first-tier stages. Individuals at each stage in this first tier of our human moral development are characterized by thinking that their way of seeing and valuing is the only correct perspective; all others are skewed. For example, a blue fundamentalist will despise an orange rationalist or sensitive green environmentalist and believe they are both going to hell. The orange will consider the blue to be a nutcase Bible thumper and the green to be a weak-minded tree hugger; the green will agree with the orange about the blue, but consider the orange to be a Gaia-wrecking, greedy capitalist. In short, first tier is a food fight with all of these levels seeking dominance over the others. In the United States, we call this fight for dominance "culture wars."

What also occurs at first-tier stages is often a partial or sometimes complete dissociation from the prior stage of development as one grows into a new stage. This is normal and even necessary in the beginning. But it becomes a problem when the goodness and strengths of prior levels are left behind, the babies along with the bathwater. A newly emergent orange seldom takes the good aspects of blue along for the journey into orange, namely the humility and orientation towards service and community. Unhealthy orange is, in fact, often characterized by extreme individualism, greed, and an "I got mine; too bad about you" attitude. Green will often reject the great gifts of orange as poisoned fruits of greedy capitalism, not understanding that the technological inventiveness of orange is what allowed green to emerge in the first place. Think of the conversations that happen around the dinner table when families get together during the holidays. One could unpack this problem of the first-tier food fight in a thousand different ways, but as soon as one internalizes Spiral Dynamics on an individual level, or on the level of how humans develop in general, many things become understandable, if not easily fixable, and begin to fall into place.

If the story ended here, we would be in deep trouble, which in fact we are. But happily, as I have said before, "Stress is the mother of evolution." Because of first-tier chaos, something new is beginning to emerge on the horizon—something that is shedding light on a seemingly hopeless situation. What begins to happen at second tier is a healthy developmental growth characterized by transcending and *including* the stage that went before. As Harvard psychologist Robert Kegan says, the subject of one developmental level becomes the object of the next.[11] In Integral Recovery terms, this is represented by the shift from "I am an addict" to "I have an addiction." The formerly in-control addict self is no longer the "I" who is calling the shots, but has now becomes a "mine"—something to own and do one's best to deal with responsibly. The controlling subject, at the altitude where the addiction once found its center of gravity, now becomes the object of the next developmental stage in the recovery process.

Second Tier

Transcendence, inclusion, and healing of first-tier stages of development are the tasks of second tier, where we can assimilate and metabolize all the strengths and gifts offered by each and every one of the prior stages. Ultimately, this includes forgiveness and reconciliation between the different stages of development. At first tier, the preceding stages and their failings and internal contradictions are often used as the foil, motivator, or raw material with which to build the next stage of development. And because there is often flack and attacks from the members of the stage one is leaving behind, the relationship with the prior stage is often adversarial and antagonistic. For example, if one were to stand up in a conservative Christian Church and say, "My dear friends, I love you, and the last thirty years have been great, but I now feel called to go study Buddhism," well, you can imagine the reaction!

It is, therefore, in large part up to second tier to heal these divisions and dissociations and to work toward allowing developmental transitions to actually become inclusive and respectful of prior stages so that each new stage is ever more healthy than the last and no longer seen as threatening by those currently at a lower stage of development. This, I feel, is one of the great promises of Integral awareness, or second tier, as it begins to come online more fully within the human family. The agenda or mission of second tier is not so much to promote second-tier thinking, but to work toward the healthy expression of first tier, since this is where most of humanity currently resides and will continue to dwell for the foreseeable future.

Einstein once said that a problem could not be solved on the level it was created—just as in Spiral Dynamics, the problems and challenges that are created at one stage of development are only truly resolved and effectively addressed at the next stage of evolutionary growth. The stress, crises, and chaos created at one level become the creative matrix out of which the next higher level of development emerges. In the case of addiction, the dragons, the overpowering cravings for drugs, become objects that arise in a context of expanded awareness. Only now can they be assimilated, transformed, and released and are no longer the controlling demons of one's existence. In fact, without these dragons of chaos, crisis, and stress, there would be little higher-order development or growth.[12] As we move from being the controlled prisoner of our cravings to the enlightened Witness, we progressively become freer of our chains and compulsions. This process is the "up-leveling" Einstein was speaking of on the level of the human spirit.

**The United States:
Predominant Levels in U.S. Culture (Where We Are At)**

It's important to understand that Spiral Dynamics does not describe levels of people, but rather levels within people. We can all pass through (and retain access to) all of these levels as we grow and evolve through life. We know that red is concerned with regaining autonomy and honor; blue with forgiveness and aligning oneself with one's Higher Power, or God's will; orange with winning and actualizing one's full potential; and green with restoring one's healthful place in the community of life.

That said, here are some general examples of these levels in the world around us.[16] In the U.S., around 20 percent of the population is said to be at blue; while predominant center of gravity is orange (around 50 percent). This puts modern green at around 20 percent. That leaves a few points for red and below and 2 to 3 percent for emergent second tier. It is also estimated that about 30 percent of green is what is called "exit green." In other words, people who have done green for a while and are starting to find it a cul de sac, insufficient to answer their needs (or the world's for that matter). This means that in the next few years, we could see rapid growth in the ranks of people arriving at Integral second-tier levels of development. In Spiral Dynamics, it is said that when 10 percent of a population arrives at the next emergent level of development, it is a "tipping" point and major shifts occur in culture and society as a whole. These next few years could get very exciting with a second-tier unfolding, and I believe Integral Recovery will play a significant role.

At each stage of development, we must balance all four quadrants and work the four essential lines or human capacities: body, mind, heart, and soul. At second tier, we work to create structures and conditions that will allow the health of the entire spiral and facilitate growth to the highest levels that individuals and cultures want and are capable of reaching. One might complain this is rather elitist, but it is an elitism to which all are invited. What we begin to understand at second tier is that we have to approach each level of development in terms that it can understand. This is done in the spirit of wisdom and compassion.

Here is an example of how a second-tier perspective can overcome the problems of a first-tier approach. Ken Wilber recorded a dialogue with a father, referring to the book *The War against Boys*,[13] which does a

The Players and the Values They Represent

Red is an impulsive/egocentric structure, mostly seen in street and prison gangs, such as Crips, Bloods, Aryan Brotherhood, Norteños, Sudeños, etc.

Blue is a traditionalist/absolutistic/mythic structure, seen in fundamentalism, xenophobic patriotism, "law and order" advocates, the "moral majority," and the evangelical movement. On the positive side, blue can also be humble, even saintly, deeply understanding the need for self sacrifice and putting the higher good or Higher Power first.

Orange is a modern/rationalist structure, emphasizing individualism and personal freedom, science and technology, achievement and success (often materialistic); it's mostly seen in the scientific paradigm, corporate culture, and free market ideology.

Green is a postmodern/pluralistic structure, seen in the sixties counterculture, the environmental movement, civil rights (including feminism and gay rights, basically everyone's rights), postmodernism, diversity and multiculturalism, political correctness, human rights advocacy, and the New Age.

"Second tier"—which indicates a "momentous leap" into a higher order of functioning—includes yellow and turquoise, and is characterized by Integral and holistic thinking, and an understanding that all previous level are necessary parts of the human evolutionary spiral. It acts *on behalf of the entire spiral*, rather than only its particular level and concerns.

Currently in the U.S., it is estimated that 20+ percent of the population is blue, 50 percent orange, 20 percent green, and only 2–3 percent second tier. On the world stage, 70 percent of the population is at the blue level or below.

brilliant job of unpacking the problem of green parents trying to impose their values on healthy, red little boys by not allowing them to play their very stage-appropriate games of soldiers, cowboys and Indians, and the like. This turns out to be a very *un*healthy repression of natural male aggression, as play-acting is a very positive way for this energy to be incorporated and released. If this red stage is not allowed to be worked out as a game or fantasy, it might be acted out later in life in ways that are dangerous and harmful, such as gang violence.

In the dialogue, the father explains how he taught his five-year-old son with ADD to meditate, using the example of how Spider Man can sit still for hours on end in order to watch the bad guys. Very effectively, this man taught his son how to meditate using language that totally resonated with where the boy was at developmentally. This is a beautiful example of Integral awareness in practice.

On a larger scale, let us take the issue of environmentalism. One can present blue with all the massive amounts of scientific data available—global warming, melting ice caps, depleted top soil, polluted and dying oceans—and they just won't hear it. Blue is prerational. You could argue science and data until you were blue in the face (pun intended). Blue is simply not there yet. In fact, they will be annoyed. But if you show them a few verses from the Bible (or whatever sacred text they adhere to) and talk to them in terms of desecrating Creation as tantamount to disrespecting the Creator, you will get their attention. At this point, you could say something like, "Let's pray together and ask for guidance and help to be better stewards of our Lord's creation." You will find this gets remarkable results, and you may start seeing real changes. This may be difficult to pull off if you are attempting it from an orange or green level because blue might detect your insincerity or discomfort. But, at second tier, the move is possible because you understand and are in touch with your own blue structure, and you can speak honestly through that part of yourself, while at the same time maintaining your second-tier perspective.

Continuing to use the environmental issue to illustrate the advantages of a second-tier perspective, when speaking about the environment to an orange person or group, you might say something like, "The numbers show that 70 percent of the population believes we are in the middle of an environmental crisis. If you make a sustainable product, you will gain X amount of market share in the short term, and in the long term, the projections look like this." They will say, "Let us see those numbers!" and you have them. To green, all you have to say is, "Trees are people too," and you have them. It is preaching to the choir. To red, the appeal is, "Cut down that tree and you'll be doing hard time!" Another, more positive, approach with red would be to say, "The wild lands need your protection; we need your courage and strength to be a protector, so here are your uniform and weapons." Give red an opportunity to be honored and respected. Another cogent argument in regard to wilderness protection for red would be: "We need the wild places because this is where to go to become men." Bring forth the positive aspects of each stage and thereby neutralize the negative aspects.[14]

As I mentioned earlier, one of the problems with first-tier development is that there seems to be an unhealthy disassociation from prior levels, and many of the strengths and gifts of preceding levels are left behind. Although negation of the prior level is often a necessary catalyst to energize the leap to the next level, this may then be experienced as a death and rebirth and can be quite painful. For example, when one is leaving a mythic, absolutist religious structure (internally) and an organization (externally), it can really be a mixed bag. On the one hand, there may be a sense of liberation and freedom, and, on the other hand, there may be a sense of dread and disorientation, because when one leaves the controlling system behind, the old certainties are left behind as well. This alone can make the leap in perspective too frightening for many.

Higher Stages: Greater Abilities and More Complex Pathologies

It should be noted that while our capacities, embrace, and complexity increase at each subsequent higher stage of development, so do the complexities of our associated pathologies. For example, I have often said somewhat jokingly, "There is nothing worse than a really smart addict," meaning that the capacity to rationalize and justify the continued use of the desired substance(s) increases as our brilliant addict spins impressive, epic, and even noble reasons to continue down the road of addiction. Again, this is simply the clever and inventive neocortex serving the primitive, overpowering cravings of the reptilian brainstem. This is an example of a high cognitive level development serving a very low moral level of development, all of which are being perverted and controlled by the progression of the disease of addiction.

Again, there is a continuous process of death to the old ideas and assumptions and a rebirth into a higher, freer, larger view or perspective. This is one of the great breakthroughs of second tier: the realization that all of our views are relative and depend on the altitude of our present developmental stage. This is not relative in the sense that all views are equal. All views are and were adequate for the challenges they needed to face, but the higher one climbs the ladder, the larger the view becomes, which broadens the perspectives one can take. This allows each higher stage to become, in a very real sense, more adequate.

Here, I would like to say that on the Integral Recovery journey it is very important to make friends with the transformational process itself. Because of the powerful synergistic effects of your IRP, and the accelerated transformational potential of meditation assisted by brainwave entrainment, transformational breakthroughs may happen quite regularly. Let us state, too, that it is the right of every human being not to transform. As one student asked me, "John, what if I want to stay blue?" The answer is, of course, that you have every right to remain blue.

Although we are not absolutely sure what causes stage growth or the transformational leap, the inner pressure or overload that throws one into chaos and upheaval tends to be characterized by dissatisfaction with and exhaustion of the present stage (at least in the case of the suffering addict). As they say in AA, "Sick and tired of being sick and tired." At the same time, there is an attraction to the prospect of growth to the next higher available stage and beyond. All stage growth, spiritual growth, or "escaping into higher order"[15] is chaotic and can feel terrifying if one does not know what is going on. Can you imagine the terror of giving birth if you did not know what was happening? It would seem that that you were being destroyed and ripped apart from the inside, instead of bringing forth new life. However, if one understands the process of birth and is prepared for it, it can be one of the most spiritual experiences available to human beings. So it is essential for skillful, conscious growth and evolution that we understand that practice can, and often should, be a process whereby we let the inner pressure increase, and not release it or run from it, because chaos and upheaval are truly the mothers of transformation and evolution.

This is a point that cannot be stressed enough, because early recovery can often be chaotic, and I believe it is often the fear of chaos itself that leads the addict to use drugs in the first place. As we learn to embrace chaos as friend, teacher, and transformational principle of the universe—from chemical reactions, to the human brain, to the evolution of life and consciousness itself—as we welcome and in some sense allow the changes to occur in us, we become not only vehicles of the evolutionary process, but conscious participants in our own evolution. This is exciting new ground for humanity as a whole and recovery specifically.

This developmental dimension is what adds such an important evolutionary perspective to Integral Recovery and puts it in a class by itself as far as the recovery world is concerned. To put it simply, Integral Recovery is a second-tier approach to treatment, in a world where the cutting edge to this point has been green. Passing the Rubicon into second tier has been likened to becoming a cube in a land of squares. Once Spiral Dynamics has been grasped and understood, one can't just go back to seeing things in the same old first-tier way. Once we can perceive the problem from a second-tier altitude, then the challenge becomes to bring our skill level up to our ability to perceive. In Integral Recovery, this means that we must learn to meet our clients where they are at, framing and individualizing our treatment modalities to meet the client's particular developmental needs. Balancing the quadrants and the five essential lines is the key to recovery and health at any level, but how those are taught and approached must be adapted to the altitude of the client.

Spiral Dynamics and Alcoholics Anonymous

Alcoholics Anonymous and related 12-step groups are enormously important. They have dominated the field of recovery for the last fifty years. It is useful to apply the Integral map to our understanding of AA, and specifically the lens of Spiral Dynamics, to help us understand AA at a deeper level—understand its successes and failures, using our knowledge of vertical developmental structures. As it is popularly practiced and interpreted, AA is largely a blue-meme organization. That does not mean that Bill W.'s original inspiration was not worldcentric orange, or even higher, in some aspects. "A God of your understanding" is not a blue (traditionalist) concept—it is much broader than that. And the self-governing, egalitarian traditions of AA are not conformist in a blue sense. But many of the AA Lower-Left quadrant cultural beliefs and practices are blue to the core. These include the centrality of the sacred text (*Big Book*), which is seen by many as inspired and virtually infallible; the mythic membership culture ("us" alcoholics as opposed to the "normies"); the distrust of science and "experts"; and the fact that there is no easy or honorable way to leave the fellowship of AA. Leaving AA or the group is generally considered the equivalent of relapse or backsliding in many 12-step groups.

These blue cultural aspects of AA are a turn off to many therapists, as well as addicts, who have a center of gravity at orange, green, or higher. But the good news is that many of these issues could be overcome quite gracefully if AA would become more Integrally informed and begin to support growth into orange, green, and higher levels of development. In other words, we could transcend and include the positive aspects of AA—the spirituality, the sense of fellowship, the ethic of service—in a more Integral approach. Healthy developmental growth means preserving the baby at each developmental level, while throwing out the bathwater that is no longer appropriate or useful as we move to our next stage of development. The bathwater, however, should also be honored, because it, or the inadequacies of each prior level, is what has provided the drive and the fuel to continue the journey of growth and transcendence. This is one reason why working with addicts can be so exciting and rewarding: the egocentric addict stage has just become so bloody awful, unacceptable, and deadly that the existential given becomes, "Evolve or die!" The work of healing and growing is not a lifestyle choice but a survival imperative.

4

Working the Lines

In Integral Recovery, sobriety is only first base. Home plate is balance
in all four quadrants and mastery in all essential lines.

—John Dupuy

The third component of our AQAL map, after quadrants and levels, is
lines. The idea of lines, or multiple intelligences, first came onto the popular scene with Howard Gardner's work, *The Theory of Multiple Intelligences*.[1]
Lines are individual, semi-independent human capacities or intelligences,
such as cognitive intelligence, spiritual intelligence, emotional intelligence,
kinesthetic (body) intelligence, mathematical intelligence, musical intelligence, and so on. We call them lines instead of just intelligences, because
lines give us a way to measure them against each other on a vertical
scale. For example, someone could be very developed cognitively (have
a high I.Q.), and extremely dumb emotionally (I think we've all known
people like this). The fact that we could be highly developed in some
aspects of our lives and underdeveloped in others is usually intuitive and
immediately graspable to most of us.

In Integral assessment, we often use a psychograph to illustrate how
these different capacities and intelligences stand in relationship to one
another. The five main lines that we normally deal with are (1) spiritual,
(2) emotional, (3) cognitive, (4) physical, and (5) ethical.[2] These lines can
easily be visualized and used as a method to examine our Integral health.
For example, a person might be highly developed cognitively, but very
low physically (in terrible shape), with a very low spiritual intelligence,
midrange emotional intelligence, and practically no ethical intelligence. It
would be easy to understand that this person is in big trouble, as a very
intelligent person with no ethics and some emotional intelligence can

do a lot of damage to himself and others. A good example, which Ken Wilber often uses, are the Nazi doctors who performed experiments on prisoners in concentration camps. They might have been very intelligent cognitively, but absolute cretins ethically and morally. As a consequence of their lines configuration, they may cause great harm to others and ultimately to themselves.

There are various ways of determining an individual's psychograph. It can be determined intuitively, which becomes a valuable self-evaluation tool. Most of us, if we look at ourselves honestly, could create a fairly accurate psychograph within a very short time. For a counselor or a therapist, it is not difficult to come up with a working psychograph based on interviews and consultations with a student or client. Actual tests are also being developed within the Integral community.[3]

Using lines as a map and a guide, we can see that for Integral health and Integral recovery we will need to push the essential lines at least into a healthy and balanced range. Based on the work of George Leonard and Michael Murphy,[4] and later Ken Wilber and the Integral Institute,[5] in Integral Recovery, we have selected five of these intelligences, human capacities, or lines, to be the centerpiece of our IRP. These five lines, body, mind, spirit, emotions, and ethics, are what we call the essential self-related lines. This means that if you're pathologically deficient in any one of these essential lines, your health, self, and sobriety will suffer. Other lines that are nonessential, such as musical or culinary lines, might be nice to develop, but they are not judged as essential unless you are a chef or a professional musician, if you get my drift.

The Cognitive Line

Interestingly, we find that it is usually the cognitive line that leads the way in raising all of the lines. In Integral Recovery, we begin working with our cognitive line by learning the scientific basis of the disease of addiction and the basics of the AQAL map. This gives us a new way to understand and explore the world and our experience—an important first step. We learn why Integral is such an invaluable theoretical framework and what Integral health might look like for us. With these intellectual understandings, we can then begin to implement our practices and take the steps necessary to achieve optimal health in all of the essential lines. Another aspect of cognitive growth, one of the touchstones of Integral

Recovery, is the fact that cognitive intelligence, as it grows, is not just about number crunching and data processing, but, even more importantly, includes the ability to take other perspectives beyond our own. As I said earlier, at the pathological, egocentric level of the addict, in the latter progression of the disease, there is only one perspective available, namely the addicted self. As addicts, when we begin to heal, the first step is moving from egocentric to ethnocentric, where we start to realize that we are not an island and that our disease and the misdeeds caused by this condition have not only hurt us but have caused great suffering and pain to those around us.

In Integral Recovery, we believe that a stable, healthy, ethnocentric level of moral and cognitive development is foundational to sustain sobriety. It is the cognitive capacity to see ourselves through the eyes of others that brings on the moral and spiritual strength and clarity necessary to stick with the program. As I stated earlier, there is a very valid egocentric argument for recovery; namely, if I don't stop taking drugs, I will die. But the compulsivity and the "Don't tell *me* what to do!" attitude of the egocentric perspective make recovery at this level extremely doubtful, in my experience.

If we use the AQAL map to consider the commitment we must make to get sober, we can quickly see that all four quadrants of our life are infected: physical health, interior health, relational health, ethical health, and our ability to function in the world in a meaningful way. We begin to understand the devolution of our moral development brought about by the disease, with its incessant and overpowering cravings for drugs and/or alcohol. We see how our essential human intelligences have been retarded and dragged down by the all-encompassing nature of the disease.

The Body Line

Without a healthy body as a foundation and vehicle for our minds and souls, we will greatly diminish the possibilities for the success of our higher aspirations, or lower aspirations, for that matter. (Of course, this means optimal health for *your* body, which means if you are handicapped, optimal health for your body will include the handicap.) If we have gifts to give, and we all do, they will not get to the marketplace, and they will not reach others unless our vehicle functions well enough to allow us to manifest our gifts in the world. There are also the aesthetic and personal aspects of the physical line: a strong, beautiful, and healthy body is just more pleasing, more fun, and a hell of a lot sexier. If we do not have a strong, fit body, it makes work in all the other lines more challenging and difficult, and our spiritual, emotional, and intellectual work may suffer to the point where it just doesn't happen. Once we begin to achieve a certain degree of fitness, strength, and health, it is hard to imagine ever going back to the level of illness and disease that we had before. As an old Quaker man once wrote, the key to lifelong happiness is to be a lifelong athlete.

Once the value and the ethic of rigorous exercise have been firmly implanted by virtue of our Integral practices, the change is remarkable. I cannot recall how many people over the years have profusely thanked me for inspiring them, cajoling them, and ultimately getting them to the gym, the dojo, the yoga studio. Mastering the discipline of regular exercise inevitably makes a vast difference in people's lives, their sense of self, and their level of happiness. One of the watermarks for mastery of this physical line is when we can't wait to get to the gym. We look forward to the focus, the exertion, and the "pump" from the positive neurochemicals that are released. And, frankly, it just feels good walking around in a strong, fit, well-muscled body. The idea here is not to achieve the sort of steroid-created body that one sees on the cover of *Muscle and Fitness* magazine, but simply to work out in a natural, vigorous way, producing a body with a healthy, vibrant glow of energy.

Like anything, physical exercise taken to an extreme can become counterproductive. Obsessiveness about working out can often lead to injury, as one needs to allow the body time to recover between workouts. However, the vast majority of us have not reached the point where this is a problem that we need to be concerned with. Psychiatrist and eminent author William Glasser[6] once characterized exercise as a positive addiction that everyone would do well to have.

The Emotional Line

Our emotional well-being affects every other aspect of our lives. To attain emotional health, we work on our trauma and shadow issues, which cause us pain and suffering where they reside in the basement of our unconscious. We also learn how to deal, in a healthy way, with our emotions as they arise moment to moment. Most of us have adopted unhealthy methods of dealing with our emotions, either repressing them or acting upon them in such a way as to cause harm to ourselves or others. A further aspect of emotional well-being is working with negative emotions associated with things that will happen in the future, such as our own death, the death of our loved ones, and other events perceived to be catastrophic.

We have very specific practices in our IR model to help us deal with all of these facets of emotional health. And once we begin to understand and achieve a good emotional balance, we find new freedom, energy, and creativity that spill over into all the other essential lines. Alternatively, when we are unhealthy emotionally, we are not happy; we lack creativity, spontaneity, purpose, and direction because so much of our soul and psychic energy is bound up and imprisoned in our repressed and underdeveloped emotional health.

In his recent book, *Mindsight,*[7] Dr. Daniel Siegel writes that mental illness is characterized by two qualities: rigidity and chaos. Rigidity is what happens when parts of ourselves are either compartmentalized into subpersonalities or else relegated to the basement of the unconscious. This creates a tremendous amount of problems, as so much psychic or psychological energy is required to keep these aspects of ourselves separate and repressed. Symptoms caused by this rigidity can be depression, dissociative disorders, self-destructive behaviors, hatred toward others, and, frequently, addiction and alcoholism. The second quality, chaos, is what occurs when our often tentative attempts at rigidity no longer work to control the powerful forces of the unconscious. Inner chaos can lead to bipolar depression, psychosis, and other disorders, not to mention the chaos of the latter stages of the disease of addiction.

Dr. Siegel goes on to explain that mental, emotional, and spiritual health are characterized by integration and coherence. When we begin to reown and accept the formerly compartmentalized or rejected aspects of ourselves, a new and harmonized self begins to emerge, capable of effectively integrating and transforming the many dynamic and profound aspects of our bodies, minds, and souls. That is why an Integral practice, one that covers all of the essential lines and ultimately weaves them together in a coherent, integrated whole, is an absolute necessity for Integral health and Integral recovery. A partial approach simply doesn't work and leads to pathologies, more stress, and, eventually, in the case of our addicts, relapse and death.

What we find in our brainwave entrainment enhanced meditation[8] and contemplative practices is that these rigidities and repressions begin to loosen quite rapidly and gracefully, allowing for integration and healing. That which was formerly considered the enemy, to be avoided at all costs, even to the extent of killing oneself with addictive substances, begins to be understood and accepted. The rejected part, in the words of Jesus, becomes the cornerstone of the building as well as the missing puzzle piece that allows the whole picture to come together in a more functional whole.

The Spiritual Line

The spiritual line is essential because it involves our deepest values and concerns, our very connection to our lives, our relations, the world, and the spiritual dimension, often referred to as God or Ultimate Reality. Where the spiritual line is not accounted for in a healthy way, a human being is simply deficient, or not whole. On our Integral Recovery journey, that lack of wholeness will ultimately lead to existential suffering, despair, and relapse. It is important to note that in Integral Recovery we don't present spirituality as a dogma but as an injunction. An injunction is a practice that allows us to see reality in a new way.[9]

Integral Recovery students are provided with cutting-edge techniques and technologies,[10] which allow easy, quick, and effective access to our deepest levels of consciousness, in ways that were not possible until very recently. I am constantly amazed at the depth of understanding and processing that emerges among my students, even within the first few weeks of their recovery process. With a little guidance, instruction, and 80 minutes a day (40 minutes in the morning, 40 minutes in the evening) of brainwave entrainment enhanced meditation, the changes and the realizations are striking. Sometimes it feels as if I'm talking to a group of lifelong spiritual practitioners rather than a group of people who have only been off of drugs and alcohol for a few weeks. The level of depth previously available only to the lucky few or extremely gifted has now become accessible to virtually everyone who is willing to follow the injunction to practice brainwave entrainment enhanced meditation on a daily basis.

This is the key difference between an Integral Recovery spiritual practice and a mere dogmatic buying into a set of beliefs or trying to imagine a connection with a Higher Power. We do not say, "You must believe this or that, or you will go to hell." We say, "You must look deeply within and search exhaustively—and we will give you the tools to do that." It is out of the fresh eyes provided by the new tools that a new paradigm, grounded in new data, emerges for IR practitioners. In IR, spirituality is not a practice of imagination or dogma but an actual encounter with divinity.

In Integral Recovery, we provide the technologies and techniques to look into our inner telescopes and find our deepest truths. How one approaches these truths is absolutely up to the individual. One can choose to continue in one's inherited religious tradition, such as Christianity, Judaism, Buddhism, Islam, and so on, or choose a new and independent path. No matter what direction your inner journey takes you, while exploring your deepest self, there you will find your best self. And the fruits of this journey are greater joy, peace, wisdom, purpose, and connectedness. The darkness begins to lift and we see ourselves and our world with new eyes. This is truly, I feel, one of the most remarkable and exciting aspects of Integral Recovery—that because of the technologies and techniques we have access to now, each one of us can participate in a spiritual journey of self-discovery. That which was once only available to the few has become the birthright of all of us who are willing to do the work.

Another aspect of the spiritual line is meaning. Meaning is the purpose and direction that we give to our lives and our relationships. Without a sense of meaning, our recovery, and ultimately our life, is rudderless and will almost surely crash into the rocks of "why the hell not." If we cannot answer the question, Why should we *not* take drugs? clearly and with conviction, it is highly unlikely that we will be able to maintain our sobriety, much less actualize the best version of ourselves.

As I mentioned before, when talking about the causative factors behind chronic distress, in *Man's Search for Meaning,*[11] Viktor Frankl wrote about his experiences in the Nazi death camps and how he was able to observe that those who had a reason to live and to survive were the ones who most often did. On the other hand, the prisoners who had lost their purpose and meaning often simply gave up the ghost and surrendered to death. After surviving the concentration camps, Frankl went on to form a school of existential psychology, which he called Logotherapy.[12] In Logotherapy, Dr. Frankl identifies meaning as an essential human need.

I personally feel that a large part of drug abuse and the ensuing suffering can be attributed to a lack of deep meaning and purpose in the lives of our young people. That doesn't mean that our culture today doesn't have defined meanings and purposes—albeit somewhat clichéd,

such as get a good job, get a good education, obey God, go to church,
etc.—but from the hundreds, if not thousands, of young people I have
worked with over the past few decades, I have found these particular
cultural clichés are not deeply resonant with our young people, who are
left growing up in an existential void of meaning. This leads to a narcissistic attitude like, "If it feels good and is exciting . . . why the hell not?"
Therefore, in Integral Recovery and in our spiritual work, we must ask
these questions: Why the hell shouldn't I do drugs? Why should I get
well? Our answers will often determine the outcome of our journey to
recovery.

Furthermore, our answers will continue to deepen and evolve as
we do our recovery work and IRP. At a talk I gave recently, someone
asked, "What is the meaning of life?" I was somewhat taken aback by
the question and thought of a flippant answer, but it was clear that the
person was serious and the room became silent with the spontaneous
solemnity of the moment. I answered, "The meaning of life is the meaning we give life." In other words, life is life, and as human beings, we are
the meaning givers. This meaning will deepen and broaden as we move
up the spiral from developmental stage to developmental stage. This is
not to say that we are simply inventing meaning willy-nilly, but that our
meaning creation occurs as a result of direct and meaningful encounters
with reality. As these encounters begin to include the ongoing experience
of our deepest selves, the meaning will become infused with the light of
divine wisdom and compassion.

At an ethnocentric level, meaning might come from love and loyalty
to family, and at a worldcentric level, care and concern for all peoples.
At a kosmocentric level, we get meaning from our care and concern
for all sentient beings, past, present, and future. But a crucial point here
is that this meaning quest cannot merely be a cognitive exercise, as in,
let me think about it and I'll get back to you. A mere cognitive idea
does not have the power and capacity to keep us on the path of practice, sacrifice, and transformation. While not diminishing the necessity of
the cognitive understanding, in the spiritual line in Integral Recovery,
discovery of purpose and meaning emerges—it is one of the fruits of
our inner work—and this is where we encounter the deepest, truest, and
most essential aspects of ourselves. We, as human beings, are the meaning makers of our world and when we find that meaning, we gain the
courage and understanding to reach beyond our egoic selves into the
ground of our being. This is what the spiritual line practice allows us

to achieve. This is not just a good idea, but is deemed essential, as mere self-satisfaction and narcissism does not have the depth and prerequisite strength to complete this journey.

Ethics, Morality, and Service: The Fifth Line

Being a cynic is so contemptibly easy . . . You don't have to invest anything in your work. No effort, no pride, no compassion, no sense of excellence, nothing.

—Molly Ivins

Initially, I struggled with the idea of adding ethical intelligence as a fifth line to our IRP, but over time the obviousness of its inclusion became clear. So, here it is: why, what, and how. First of all, what are ethics? And, why should we be so concerned with them that they become a central part of a lifelong practice? Simply defined, for our purposes, ethics are the moral reasons that we do what we do.

Why is ethical behavior so essential in Integral Recovery? Because unethical behavior leads to self-justification and rationalizations, which are the mother of self-deception. As Alcoholics Anonymous has long known and rightly taught, sobriety and recovery require "rigorous honesty." To be tolerated, lies and unethical behaviors become split off from the self and become festering dragons in the basement of our unconscious, where they manifest as symptoms—depression, self-hatred, hatred of others (through the process of projection), and cynicism. As our ethics and spiritual clarity are compromised, this is often followed by a "screw it all" attitude. In the recovering addict, all of these symptoms create stress in the midbrain, which, as we know, reignites the powerful craving demands of the reptile and leads to relapse and death. I don't think I am stressing this too strongly. It is essential that we embrace ethics for our spiritual health and collective long-term survival. For the recovering addict, it is a survival imperative: Do good or die! The antidote to self-deception, hypocrisy, and relapse is rigorous self-examination, practice, and ethical behavior and service.

So, how does ethics become a practice that we can work with? The first step is to dedicate our practices to the highest good we can conceive of at our current moral/ethical altitude, or center of gravity. This could look like a quiet moment before we begin a workout at the gym, where we dedicate our session to the good of our family, God, our current life's goals, the good of our human family, our planet, or whatever is most true for us. My workouts definitely take on more focus, fierceness, and intensity when I do this. A moment of dedication before we start our meditation, therapy, or cognitive or emotional releasing practices works the same way.

Here, I am reminded of the medieval story of Parsifal and the Holy Grail (not Monty Python's version). Parsifal lost the vision of the Grail and the Grail Castle when he didn't ask the right question, namely, "Whom does the Grail Serve?" Parsifal then ended up wandering around in a wasteland for many years until he found the castle again and ended up asking the right question: "Whom does the Grail serve?" The manuscript ends before he is answered, so we are left to answer the question for ourselves. Whom does our Integral Recovery Practice serve? This is the question we must ask and remind ourselves of as we do our practices. Looking and feeling good is often not enough motivation to get me to the gym or sitting on my meditation cushion, but my sense of mission and responsibility are.[13]

Ethics is an aspect of our inner meditative work, but it also necessitates behavior. For our ethics to be Integral, it must include ethical action in all four quadrants from the highest level of our current development. An IRP without ethics is foundationally weak. To choose to have an IRP is itself an ethical choice that involves all four quadrants. It is a conscious choice, at some point in the process of growth, to choose, as John Lennon said, to be part of the solution and not part of the problem. Obviously, in the first days and weeks of treatment and recovery, our motivations will be more along what Maslow referred to as "survival" needs. But for recovery to stick, a higher moral ground must be arrived at through diligence and practice. One of the signposts on this journey that we should discover through our own efforts, and heed, is that our deepest self is our highest Self.

In our quest for an active, effective, and integrating ethics and personal morality, the AQAL map is extraordinarily helpful as it allows us to act from a perspective that is high in altitude, which also covers all the essential bases. Win, win can become win, win, win . . . We make choices and act much more skillfully, in ways that not only benefit ourselves or our group, but all beings. We are more ethical in our moment-to-moment interactions, practices, and grand designs. We use the wise, compassionate

embrace of the highest levels to care for and support the healthy emergence of all stages and types in all four quadrants. The fifth line, ethics,
infuses all our practices and actions with a higher moral purpose. This
transforms our practice from narcissism to a journey of personal healing
and growth in the service of the highest good we can connect with.

How Integral Recovery Works the Lines

Understanding lines as the essential intelligences that must be cultivated
over a lifetime, through ongoing deliberate practice, becomes a loadstone
for each one of us in strengthening our recovery process and actualizing ourselves as fully developed, life-embracing, and effective human
beings. Instead of using guesswork, we can look at ourselves objectively
and form an ongoing daily and lifetime practice to achieve our goals of
optimal health and effectiveness as individuals, whatever our situations,
life tasks, and missions might be. We have learned that anything less than
this, whether we are addicts or not, leads to unnecessary wasted potential,
suffering, and, to a great extent, partially lived lives. So, what we must do
is honestly evaluate the current state of our Integral health. From that
evaluation, we can begin to implement our Integral practices and fine
tune them as we become more proficient in all the said lines.

This may sound a bit overwhelming, if not intimidating. You may
be thinking, how do I work these essential lines in a lifetime practice,
when I am already so busy as it is? To my recovery students, I say, if you
stop procuring, using, and selling drugs, you'd be amazed at how much
time is freed up. For the rest of us, it's really not so hard. Thankfully,
there is one practice in particular, the daily use of brainwave entrainment
technology (in our case, the Profound Meditation Program[14]), that actually works all five essential lines. It doesn't do everything that needs to
be done, but it works all of the lines in the following ways.

- In the physical line, brainwave entrainment (BWE) technology is actually, physically, changing our brains to work at
  ever higher levels of complexity and functionality.

- In the cognitive line, we experience a greater measure of
  cognitive capacity (we get smarter!), along with heightened
  creativity, an increase in our ability to see holistic patterns

in the massive quantities of information we are exposed to in our postmodern world, and an increased ability, over time, to take perspectives other than our own.

• In the emotional line, we experience an increased ability to handle stress, and situations and emotions that were formally overwhelming. We start to assimilate and integrate challenging emotions and traumatic material from the past much more gracefully and skillfully than before. And, as we continue with this emotional releasing and integration process, we find an ever-growing compassion for ourselves and others.

• In the spiritual line, there is a greatly increased capacity to experience deep meditational states, which leads to a greater sense of connection to our divine self and purpose, as well as an ever-deepening connection to all life and the universe. The spiritual deepening and awakening that occurs over time, when engaged in a daily BWE-enhanced meditation program, is an absolute antidote to the ever-increasing sense of isolation and despair that occurs during the progression of the disease of addiction.

• In the ethical line, and also tied into the spiritual line, we find that as our practice progresses, we develop a growing capacity to experience what many spiritual traditions call the Witness, or the Transcendent Witness. What this means is that we are able to watch ourselves from outside ourselves; instead of being lost in our traumas from the past, our conditionings, and our old dysfunctional stories, we can actually observe them from the outside. When this happens, we begin to understand that, if we can observe ourselves, or what we thought was ourselves, from outside of ourselves, then what we are must truly be greater than we formally believed we were. Over time, this witnessing happens more and more frequently, both when we are meditating and when we are not meditating.

Our Witness observes our egos and our processes with absolute equanimity and nonjudgment. To give an example, if something or someone hurts my feelings and makes me very angry, I can actually step outside of myself and witness the process of my hurt feelings and anger, my rageful and blaming thoughts. The result of witnessing in this manner is that instead of acting out on our hurt emotions, stuffing them, or numbing them with drugs, alcohol, or other dysfunctional behaviors, we can simply allow ourselves to have our thoughts and our feelings with total acceptance and understanding of them for what they are. We understand that they are not the Truth with a capital T. When we acquire this capacity, we find that our feelings, emotions, and thoughts emerge quite fully without having to be tinkered with and also that they release very quickly. After the ego storm has passed, we are often left with a deep sense of peace, even bliss, and a deeper understanding and compassion for what needs to be done—if anything—or we understand that nothing needs to be done at all.

As a result of witnessing ourselves, we are able to hold our ethics and motivations up in the light of our own internal meditative awareness. In other words, Why do I want to do a particular action? The answer might be very complex. For example, 20 percent of our motivation might be, "I want people to praise me and think I am really cool," while 40 percent might be because "I feel guilty and doing this might help assuage my guilt." The other 40 percent of our motivation might be from pure, unattached love and compassion. Just by being able to observe this, and bring this understanding forward, we can actually do the work necessary to clarify our motivations and our ethical ground. Because we are complex and not perfect, often our motivations will be less than 100 percent pure, but anything over 60 percent pure is good in my book, so carry on!

Unfortunately, there is no evidence that BWE will strengthen your bones and your muscle tissue. Alas, we still have to exercise and eat a good, healthy diet, as I like to say, lean, green, clean cuisine. But the good news is that because the BWE meditation is increasing the functioning of our brains, our workouts tend to take on a greater degree of flow and pleasure.

Finally, as we continue doing this particular practice of BWE meditation, we find we have increased our capacity for practice altogether. In other words, practice becomes easier and more natural the more we do it. And the extraordinary results that we achieve over time serve as a deep inspiration and motivation to continue the work. I have seen in myself, and over and over in my students who have used brainwave entrainment technology, that these aforementioned capacities emerge even without tutoring or coaching. However, I strongly believe that good mentoring, teaching, and coaching greatly speeds up this process.

As we work these essential lines with our practices (which we will talk more about in chapter 12), they begin to work together synergistically. The work we do in each individual line infuses the others with energy and health, allowing us to grow more quickly and more wholly. For example, as our bodies become stronger, our meditation deepens, our emotional lives becomes clearer, and our minds begin to work at a higher level.

This is the promise and the brave new world that Integral practice provides for us, and let me say emphatically that, in the IR model, these practices are not just for the addict, but for each one of us—health care providers, family members, loved ones, and so on. When all family members begin to adopt Integral practices, the whole family becomes healthier. As the Buddha indicated in his first Noble Truth, life is suffering. All of us born into this world have issues and suffer. The Integral practices outlined in this book will work equally well for all who take responsibility for their lives and practice them. Several times, I have worked with parents of an addicted child who, after a while of doing their own practices, told me, "You know, even if Billy doesn't get well, I'm going to be okay." This is a beautiful example of how Integral practices can work for all concerned. And, of course, that very attitude by the parent will facilitate the healing of the son, in this case, Billy.

Another way to use lines in an Integrally informed life is to realize your own personal strengths and weaknesses. So, for example, if you are starting a band and you are a gifted lead guitarist, you probably don't want to recruit five other gifted lead guitarists (maybe one or two). You want other musicians who do what you cannot do. Similarly, in any Integrally healthy organization, all the essential lines and intelligences necessary to accomplish our task need to be represented in order to achieve our mission in an abundantly successful way. In an un-Integral, unhealthy system, we often surround ourselves with people just like ourselves, which makes the whole venture unbalanced and unlikely to succeed. A healthy ecosystem is a diverse one.

As we continue our Integral journey to recovery and optimal health, we learn to become more skilled at recognizing which of our essential lines needs the most care and practice. What starts out as a cognitive exercise of evaluating our practice eventually becomes intuitive. We simply understand what needs to be done and where we need to ratchet it up, or perhaps we need to relax for a while. For example, it has become pretty darn clear to me at this point that when I *don't* want to meditate, this is an important indicator that I *need* to meditate. The reluctance actually signifies that there is something needing release in my consciousness that my ego doesn't want to deal with. Some days, I will intuit that today's meditation needs to be longer than an hour, as I really need more time to work on my interiors. The same is true in the realm of physical exercise—our bodies begin to sense what they need (more cardio, more yoga, less reps/more weight, less weight/more reps, etc.). Or today I need to ratchet up my mindfulness as I exercise or focus more on my breathing as I work out. The permutations and nuances are almost endless and keep our practice exciting, ever-changing, and rewarding.

I believe that personal growth in all the essential lines is a survival imperative for any addicted person. It really comes down to transcend and live or stay stuck and die. This is one of the joys of working with addicts: the "Do the work or die," no bullshit quality can be extremely clarifying as opposed to, "Well, yes, I think that meditation would be a nice addition to my lifestyle." Not that there is anything wrong with taking it easy. But there *is* something about an attitude that says, "My existence depends on my practice," that gets results and kicks the motivation to a whole new level. To both the mystic and the recovering addict, the search for God and wholeness (holiness) is an existential imperative.

At the end of chapter 1, we listed the causative factors that need to be dealt with in recovery—if recovery and sobriety are going to stick. These were:

1. Chemical imbalance in the brain

2. Unresolved trauma from the past

3. Negative narrative stories about one's self and the world

4. Inability to cope with the present

5. Lack of purpose, meaning, or connection in one's life (also known as existential despair)

6. Toxic relationships.

While we can identify these causative factors in the four quadrants, we can also see how our essential line practices address each of the factors. So, in doing our IRP, as an ongoing, lifetime commitment, we are addressing the factors that caused us to self-medicate in the first place and led to our eventual addiction. As early on, when we recognized that we were in lousy shape and really needed to get our bodies healthy and strong, when viewing our life history and emotional turmoil, we can recognize that we are sitting on a whole bunch of emotional traumas from the past, all of which need to be brought to the surface of consciousness and released, as our emotional work and meditation deepen and progress. Rather than merely being told to do a holistic hodgepodge of healthy practices, an understanding of our lines and how they relate to one another offers us an effective discipline and focused approach to deal with these causative factors.

Here, I will offer an example of how these practices of developing all of our essential lines play out in the real world. I will quote from an article I wrote recently, "Spiritual Teachers: Millstones, Responsibility, and Love."[15]

> I was attending a dinner that followed a salon on "Insight and Chaos" in Berlin, and was sitting at a table with a German man—a very accomplished Ph.D. and co-chairman of a large foundation in Germany. During our conversation, he commented that he was from Dresden, a city that had been firebombed by the allied British and American forces in WWII. I was about to make an excuse about it, which was so stupid that I won't include it here, but what I said was, "I'm sorry." He looked at me rather shocked and said, "No, no, who are we to talk," meaning the Germans, "We did so much."
>
> After the dinner was over, I took this gentleman aside and told him, "I mean it. I'm really sorry. The firebombing of Dresden was not necessary. We didn't have to do it. I'm so sorry." At this point I hugged him and kissed his neck and I'm sure my tears wet his coat, neck, and hair. He cried, too, and said, "Thank you. It means so much to me for an American to say that, and you guys have done so much good for us, but thank you." We were both profoundly moved and I immediately put on my sunglasses, as I often do when I

lose it in love, in public. Love is so often simply saying, "I'm sorry," and washing others' wounds with our tears. He that is greatest among us will be the servant of all.

After this article was published, I sent it to the gentleman who had shared the experience with me. The following is quoted from his response to me (translated from the German).

How beautiful, that you, the initiator of the gesture, experienced it equally intensely. It was a moment in which all of my arguments and opinions were rendered obsolete, and only one thing mattered: love and compassion. No need for thinking or even talking. That is what I experienced—a really spiritual moment.

Initially, as we got onto the subject of Dresden, I didn't have a reconciliation in mind at all. Rather, I wanted to argue with you, wanted to fight and win the argument, wanted to be in the right. I was even prepared to hurt you, as a representative for all Americans, if only for my pain to be recognized. What is that but to carry on the war with words?

Your "I am sorry" took away all of the aggression. It was the end of the spiral of violence, of hurt. We didn't even have to talk any more: we had understood that *Liebe und Leben*, Love and Life, come from the very same source.

A moment like this is evidence of and the foundation for the peaceful solution of all of our problems. It requires, however, that I take the first step, regardless of what type of situation it is. Here you took the first step and for that I am very grateful. The deep wound that my family had experienced was not only healed but also transformed into love.

5

Integrating Healthy States of Consciousness

States refer to the basic states of consciousness that human beings experience: waking, dreaming, and deep sleep. They also include altered and meditative states and spiritual experiences. In the Integral map, we differentiate between stages of consciousness and states of consciousness. States encompass thoughts, feelings, and experiences that arise in our awareness. They come, and they go. Feelings of happiness, for example, come and go, and trying to control these feelings to feel happy all the time is the cause of great suffering for the addict (and for everyone else). States can be glorious, awful, boring, indifferent, or anything in between.

A helpful way to think of states is, if our consciousness or pure awareness is the sky, then states are the objects that arise in the sky, such as bugs, birds, clouds, and planes. These states or objects of consciousness appear and disappear, in the context of the sky. They are ever changing. The more we understand the fleeting quality of states, the less we are slaves to them, and the more we can skillfully use them to promote healthy stage development. For example, attachment to or avoidance of certain states can keep us stuck, unhealthy, and serially relapsing. However, when approached with wisdom and skill, states can be metabolized, transmuted, released, and used as raw energy for growth, gaining wisdom, creativity, compassion, and higher stage development. For now, simply put, states are temporary states of consciousness. As Wilber has said, "States are free, stages are earned, but without states who would want stages?"[1]

States, which are some of the most intimate features of our life, are things that are seldom talked about in our flatland, scientific, academic world. But states are part of our moment-to-moment experiences of reality and are closer to us, as the Buddhist saying goes, than our own eyes. Our Integral approach to states unites the great spiritual traditions' premodern understanding of the basic states of consciousness with modern, scientific approaches.

The basic states are waking, dreaming, and deep sleep—or, to put it another way, gross, subtle, causal, and nondual. Gross states of consciousness arise and are experienced as we move through the world in a waking state. In gross, waking states, there are physical objects to bump into. Dreaming states, or subtle states of consciousness, are states that arise when we are dreaming, in REM sleep. In dreaming states, we move in a subtle form of consciousness where the "I" is still present; there are characters, feelings, emotions, and thoughts, but it is not the gross or physical realm. Any experiences or feelings that arise in this dream state are referred to as subtle experiences. We can experience subtle states during waking or gross states in what used to be called reveries, or "in our mind's eye," or waking dreams. Almost all of us can recall instances of this, and many of us remember our dreaming states (many of us do not). But we all go there every day in a 24-hour cycle (unless we are meth addicts or some other anomaly).

The next basic state is deep sleep, or the causal state. We all enter this state each night when we are in deep sleep and not dreaming. It is said that in this state of consciousness there is pure awareness. Here there are no gross objects to bump into, no objects of consciousness, not even any thoughts or subtle imagery—just pure awareness. And finally, some traditions, such as the Buddhist and the Vedantic Hindu, have identified a state beyond all states, the nondual state. The nondual state is actually not a state at all but simply the awareness in which all other states arise. The difference between the causal state and nondual is that causal is pure awareness without any objects of consciousness, and nondual includes all the states and all the objects of consciousness.

You could imagine the nondual state as the blackboard as well as what is written on the blackboard, which is all states and objects of consciousness, such as thoughts, feelings, and so on. Becoming aware of yourself as this creative context or blackboard, in which all arises moment to moment, to include the whole universe, is sometimes referred to as enlightenment. Those who can hold this awareness constantly and consistently are considered to be enlightened beings. This is important in Integral Recovery, because by doing our meditation practices, using brainwave entrainment technology, we are able to quickly access these expanded states of consciousness. When we are able to view our conditioning, our wounds, and our ego from this expanded awareness, we become free. It causes a shift in consciousness, and we begin to achieve freedom from that which was formerly a trap. This occurs in steps and stages, sometimes very dramatically and other times more subtly, but to ensure that these realizations become a permanent part of our awareness, our practice must be ongoing.

The last twenty years can be characterized as the golden age of brain research. In fact, scientists are now saying that we have learned more about the brain in the last five years than in the previous 5,000 years! As part of this ongoing revelation, scientists have found that each of these states is associated with particular brainwave frequencies. These basic brainwave frequencies are known as beta, alpha, theta, and delta. Brainwave states are recorded as waves: the waves of beta are very small and rapid; alpha waves are a little larger and a little slower; theta waves are larger and slower still; and delta waves are very large and very slow. We all experience the basic states in a normal 24-hour cycle. The wisdom traditions of the East teach about these states, and they have been confirmed by modern science.

Beta (13–30+Hz)

Beta is the state of normal, wakeful consciousness. As we are working, driving, talking, etc., we are likely in Beta. At its higher extremes, beta is sometimes associated with anxiety, panic, or stress.

Alpha (8-12.9 Hz)

Alpha is a state of light relaxation. Not a sleep state, but usually reflective of a calm, focused mind. Alpha is sometimes called the "super learning state," because the brain seems to be receptive and open to new information. Alpha is also considered ideal for creative brainstorming. Most meditation occurs in this state.

Theta (4–7.9 Hz)

Theta is a state of deep relaxation. Sometimes a sleep state, sometimes not, theta reflects a state of dreamlike awareness. Dreams and a deep, meditative state of consciousness are common characteristics of theta.

Delta (0.1–3.9 Hz)

Delta, the deepest of the brainwave patterns, is a state of deep sleep, or trance-like consciousness. This state of dreamless sleep or pure consciousness is without objects; there is awareness, but no thoughts, feelings, emotions, etc. Maintaining awareness into delta can result in accessing the unconscious portion of our consciousness.

After Delta, the traditions teach us there is the Transcendent Witness—the pure open spaciousness in which all these other realms arise.

Figure 6. Brainwave States

Beta waves are associated with waking consciousness or gross states. These very rapid waves correspond to our day-to-day thinking processes, which in most cases are quite cluttered. Buddhists call this "monkey mind." Alpha waves are also associated with waking consciousness, but alpha is a brainwave state that is predominant when we are very focused and concentrated, such as when we are totally engrossed in reading a book to the exclusion of all that is going on around us. Theta is the brainwave state that is associated with subtle or dream states. In this brainwave state, we move through an imaginary, subtle universe. And delta waves correspond with the deepest, dreamless states of consciousness, causal and nondual.

What, you might ask, does this have to do with Integral Recovery? Actually, an enormous amount. In the early 1970s, scientists learned that skillful meditators could alter their brainwave states through their meditative practices. Frequently, these meditators could change their brainwave states from beta to alpha and at times could spike down briefly into theta. Meditators who could do this reported that the positive fruits of their meditative practice were increased concentration, greater serenity, and feelings of bliss. The scientists also noted that these practitioners could lower their blood pressure at will and achieve other salutary effects through their meditative practices.

In the late 1970s, it was discovered that deep meditative brainwave states could be achieved relatively quickly through binaural means.[2] This greatly expanded the horizons of what was possible to achieve with the human brain. In other words, deep meditation became a potential for everyone and not just the few who had the skill and time to develop a disciplined practice. Binaural brainwave entrainment makes the fruits of a deep monastic meditative practice available to anyone who does the binaural practices.

In the early days of binaural brainwave entrainment, it was thought that the ideal meditative brainwave state was alpha and that this brainwave state was the level where "superlearning" occurs. Subsequently, for some time, theta was thought to be the ideal level to entrain brain waves to, and, more recently, it was found that the deepest and the slowest brain wavelength, delta, is the most powerful for deep meditation, healing, and transformation.[3]

Our knowledge of states and brain waves and our ability to entrain the brain are perhaps some of the most exciting and positive discoveries of the twentieth century and are only now starting to be put to use by a significant amount of people. This knowledge gives us a new understanding of our own awareness, moment to moment, how our brains function, and how we can use this knowledge and the technologies that have become available to us to deepen our emotional lives and understanding, to awaken our spiritual natures, and to increase our cognitive abilities in ways that were never before possible. In the case of Integral Recovery, it is truly epoch making in its ability to heal, rebalance, and transform the brain, attacking the disease of addiction where it lives (in the human brain).

I have found the states aspect of the AQAL map to be a very easy sell with addicts, because if there is one thing that a drug or alcohol user knows, it's states of consciousness. They have *lived* for these altered states: a shot of tequila, a line of coke, an injection of heroin, and presto! You have an altered state. In fact, drug addiction could be defined as a compulsive attachment to certain states brought about by the drug(s) of choice. The other side of that coin is eschewing other states of consciousness such as anxiety, depression, and the feelings that accompany withdrawal. Either of these strategies, the grasping onto that which is desired or the pushing away of that which is not, lead to the same thing, namely, suffering and dysfunction. The "big lie," the sirens' song of addiction, is that by using you won't have to suffer all the foibles of life anymore. You can just keep altering and altering and altering your consciousness (states) until well . . . there's nothing left to alter. The promise of escape from suffering is, at bottom, a twisted justification on the part of the neocortex for giving in to all of the controlling demands coming from the reptilian brain.

I've often asked students why they started using drugs in the first place, and I've received all kinds of answers, such as to escape anxiety, to lessen depression, to feel good, to find some peace, to feel at home in my own skin, to have fun, and so on. Then I ask, "What did you end up with?" The most common response is, "F——ing hell." At this point, I explain, "You were chasing states. This in itself is not bad; you were just doing it the wrong way." We need to learn to master our states and not to become their slaves.

One of the great fears of those beginning the process of recovery is that they will never be able to experience pleasure again. When newly recovering addicts realize that they will still be able to achieve experiences of bliss and ecstasy that are not unhealthy and drug dependent, but are actually an essential part of their lives and IRP, there is a great sense of relief. David Deida, spiritual teacher,[4] has drawn a useful distinction between endogenous states of consciousness, proceeding from within, and exogenous states of consciousness, proceeding from outside.[5] Exogenous states of consciousness are states achieved by using things such as drugs. While these states are very powerful, they unfortunately do not lead to stage growth. For example, you could use LSD every week for thirty years and not experience any stage growth. However, endogenous states of consciousness are states achieved through meditation and other practices. These actually lead to higher stages of consciousness, which is one of the primary goals of Integral Recovery.

Deep states of consciousness, such as those we access in meditation using brainwave entrainment technology, essentially metabolize over time and begin to create the actual structures of higher stage development. Our goal is to reach those higher stages of consciousness where "I am an addict" transcends to "I have an addiction." As we said earlier, in our chapter on stages, it seems hard for recovery to stick at very low ego-centric levels of development. So higher-stage development is intrinsic to our quest for Integral Recovery. In our meditation, we also have access to our "emergent self." In other words, we are able to glimpse previews of our possible future stage development. Wilber has said, in various talks, and this has certainly been confirmed in my work, that one encounters three things in deep meditative practice: (1) the submerged self, leftover trauma and business from the past, (2) our present developmental stage, and (3) our future or emergent self. And it is this contact with our future or emergent possibilities that often fuels our meditative practice with the inspiration to stick with it. As mentioned earlier, without these inspiring previews, we probably would not stick around to do the necessary work.

In Integral Recovery, we learn to understand all types of states of consciousness: meditative states, contemplative states, drug-induced states, and normal states, such as happiness, fear, and anxiety. Learning that states are just the foreground noise that comes and goes causes a huge shift in our relationship to reality and how it is experienced and processed. As we deepen our meditative practice, we begin to identify more with pure consciousness itself, our context, and identify less with the objects that come and go, our content. And when we do this on a regular basis, we wind up living the content of our lives with much greater freedom, clarity, and effectiveness.

When we are too caught up in the stories or content of our life (as we commonly are), we become slaves to our past, our conditioning, and our current state of consciousness. We react instead of act. However, as we become more identified with pure awareness or spaciousness as our true, enduring, essential nature, we become more enlightened, or, in the words of Roger Walsh,[6] more spiritually mature. This understanding of states of consciousness versus pure consciousness can come in an intuitive flash of knowing and then our ongoing practice deepens and stabilizes this knowledge.

Early on in my own pioneering efforts with an IRP, I encountered the Sedona Method,[7] Buddhist teachings, and Ken Wilber's writings about states versus stages. Synthesizing these three into a working knowledge of states quickly became a very important understanding for my own practice, as well as for those with whom I subsequently worked. I found that in deep, BWE-enhanced meditative states, I could get in touch with many states and feelings that I had formerly repressed, sometimes consciously, sometimes not. Over time, I was able to allow these states of consciousness to arise and then release them. This was extremely healing for me, as many of these repressed states and feelings had been causing me suffering, depression, and illness for years. As well as learning to skillfully deal with many varied states of consciousness, from absolute bliss and peace to darkest despair, I soon became aware that there was something even deeper and more basic than these states themselves. This was the pure consciousness, or awareness, in which all states arise.

The Wilber-Combs lattice is a major contribution of Ken Wilber and Allan Combs to our understanding of states versus stages. It postulates that one can have any state of consciousness at any *stage* of consciousness. This means, for example, that if one has a major spiritual experience at, say, a blue mythic stage of consciousness, one will interpret that state of consciousness through the tools and perspectives that are available at a blue stage of consciousness. This is a hugely important understanding in spiritual practice and psychology, because it helps us to understand that even though we can change our states of consciousness using the many technologies now available, it is really our stage of consciousness that determines our interpretation of what those states mean to us. Depending on our stage, we might have a relatively more useful and compassionate interpretation of our current state. For example, a depressed person whose center of gravity is egocentric red will experience and interpret a depressed state very differently from a depressed person at a worldcentric orange stage of development.

At red, a spiritual experience of higher consciousness or God is interpreted purely on egocentric terms: Jesus came to me, or I am Jesus. At blue, because of the absolutistic nature of blue, the interpretation might be, this is the Truth (for everyone). At orange, we might interpret our

experience scientifically and compare it with experiences from traditions
other than our own. At green, our experience is likely to be interpreted
in terms of universal love and acceptance of all beings and traditions. And,
at second tier, we bring an Integral analysis to our experience, which
affects its usefulness, meaning, and overall effect on us. As Wilber has
often said, the experience is not nearly as important as how we interpret
it and what we do with it.

Perhaps what is most important is that in our Integral Recovery
Practice we learn that states are temporary and are something to be
worked with as we accept, feel, and release them; in this way they become
the raw materials of our healing, promoting healthy current-stage development and growth. A major part of the genius of the AQAL model is
that it shines a light on the states that have to do with our experience
of being alive moment to moment, allowing us to both understand them
at a deeper level and to work with them effectively. Just being aware of
states in this conversation, for example, is a mini-transcendent experience,
at least intellectually. As we learn, we begin to see states as something
outside of our essential self. Even this small bit of disidentification from
states can offer us a taste of freedom from them. We learn to accept and
experience states fully, but at the same time not be their slaves. Most of
our unconscious patterns in dealing with states involve trying to achieve
certain states, such as happiness or romantic love, and avoid others, such
as sadness, depression, anxiety, boredom, and loneliness.

Normally, there are three things we tend to do with states. In the
case of positive states, we try to hold on to them because they feel so
good. In the case of negative states, we attempt to repress them because
they are unacceptable or too scary. Or we project our unwanted feelings
on others and blame them as the source. In the case of addiction, there is
of course another method of dealing with states, which is to narcoticize
ourselves in an attempt to always feel good and never feel bad or never
have to feel at all. All of these strategies are somewhat successful in the
short term, but leave us dissociated and unhealthy in the long term. In
our Integral Recovery Practice, we learn to allow states of consciousness
to arise, and we even invite them in. Sometimes, during my meditation, I will ask myself, "Is there anything I need to look at that I have
been avoiding?" We learn to let our different states arise naturally in
our practice and in our lives, as their repression and avoidance can lead
to a variety of pathological consequences. We also learn to not become
attached even to our desirable states.

States or feelings that arise from our unconscious minds could be happiness or bliss; it is not always the negative ones that we repress. Sometimes we are afraid of our joy, as suggested in the title of C. S. Lewis' beautiful memoir, *Surprised by Joy*. We may avoid pleasant states such as those associated with pride and self-esteem. We can imagine Eeyore, the beloved donkey from *Winnie the Pooh*, having a problem accepting states that induce joy and hope. So, whether we are gloomy Eeyores, Sevens on the Enneagram,[8] or another sort who is only attracted to states of happiness, we must learn to accept and fully experience the multitude of states that arise in our consciousness moment to moment and not attach unmerited importance to whatever states arise. After all, they are just states! And they come and go. In the immortal words of Stuart Davis, Integral rock star, "Never trust a state." Or, as a student of mine once told me, "Don't make a philosophy out of it [the state]!"[9]

In our meditation, we can learn to identify with the Witness, sometimes called the Transcendent Witness, who simply watches all of our various states arise without judgment or attachment, perhaps with profound curiosity, like a scientist in the Amazon who has just encountered a rare flower or a butterfly. Then we simply allow the state of consciousness, emotion, or feeling to do whatever it needs to do to be fully accepted, experienced, and thereby released. Most often, we will begin to feel it somewhere in our body, our gut, our heart, or our head. As my friend and teacher Christian Meyer told me once, "You don't have to do anything with feelings; just let the feelings do whatever they want with you." So, if the feeling arising is grief, for example, we would let the grief be felt completely in our bodies (often our heart) and let that grief control our breathing, where it might become sobbing or some other manifestation of grief. By allowing the feeling or state to fully express itself, without control or interpretation, we find that it soon passes, and in its wake, we are left with a profound sense of spaciousness, peace, and inner depth. In that place, which is beyond states, we begin to explore and understand the mystery that has always been a part of humanity's quest since we became self-reflective, which is, namely, Who am I?

In the beginning, this type of work may seem difficult and even scary. But as we mature and become masters of our inner work, this becomes second nature. We can do this while we are doing our meditation, on a bus going to work, or in a conversation with a friend. As we continue to practice this ability to be open, witnessing what arises and allowing our feelings to be felt, we not only become free of our past, but we also become free in the present. And, as with all of our practices, it gets easier and deeply more satisfying with time and daily effort. Our practice progresses from "I need to do this," to "I want to do this," to "I like to do this," to "This is just what I do."

So, as we can see, an intellectual understanding of states as illuminated by the AQAL model, along with a practical, contemplative, and meditative understanding of how to work with them can become a doorway to profound healing, liberation, and emotional and spiritual maturity. It brings about an extraordinary deepening of spiritual and emotional life, as well as a transcendently new way to approach recovery and spiritual and emotional healing.

6

Understanding Types

What are types, and why are types important to our Integral Recovery process? The last essential lens of the AQAL map is called types. Types represent the basic personality styles or orientations, such as masculine/feminine, and personality types as elucidated in typologies like the Enneagram and Myers-Briggs. Types provide us with several very useful perspectives, which enable us to understand individuals more skillfully and with greater wisdom and insight. Ultimately, they allow us to be more effective and compassionate with ourselves and others. Another real plus to including types in a map of human experience is that we learn that there are many strategies and ways of coping (or not coping) and healing, depending on one's typology and orientation.

In addiction treatment, one's type can have a great deal to do with how and why one started using drugs in the first place and also (perhaps this needs more study) which drug one chooses according to one's personality type and emotional issues and deficits. Through types, we learn what our particular traps are and the ways out of these traps. For example, using the AQAL map, we could look at another individual, or ourselves, and say, "Bob is a masculine-identified Eight on the Enneagram, whose center of gravity is orange." Right off, this gives us a tremendous amount of information, and from there we can move on to a complete AQAL analysis, such as what is going on in the four quadrants of his life and how he is doing in his five essential lines, body, mind, heart, soul, and ethics. Already, we have enough questions, and hopefully information, to afford us a truly Integral and effective strategy to deal with Bob and help Bob to deal with and heal himself and his life.

I, personally, am a Six on the Enneagram, and there are certain things I have to confront on my healing journey because of that, but they are not necessarily the same things that, say, a Seven on the Enneagram might need to deal with or should deal with in the same way. Often, I have found that nonintegral healers, counselors, and therapists will find something that worked for them and think it is a solution for everyone. As we understand types more thoroughly, other types as well as our own, we will avoid cookie-cutter approaches and move skillfully in the process and flow of healing and awakening with the effortless grace of the master of aikido, using the very ego structures and energies in the evolutionary unfolding that is Integral Recovery.

Integrating Masculine and Feminine

The first two basic types that we identify are masculine and feminine. Notice I did not say male and female, as all individuals have masculine and feminine aspects regardless of their gender. In general, we say that the masculine tends toward exterior accomplishment, achievement, and goal-oriented activity. The feminine tends toward relationship and communion. Masculine pathology tends toward narcissistic achievement regardless of its effects on others, and feminine pathology tends toward losing oneself unhealthily in relationships. In order to heal, the masculine needs the feminine quality of caring and relationship, and the feminine needs the masculine strength of autonomy, personal boundary setting, and self-reliance.

In the case of addiction, the pathological aspects of masculine and feminine play themselves out with the unhealthy masculine using drugs for control and the unhealthy feminine using drugs for comfort and escape. For recovery to be effective, the addict must reclaim and balance the healthy aspects of both feminine and masculine: the ability to assert masculine willpower, and the ability to care for others in a healthy, nourishing way.

Carl Jung taught that in order for the male aspect of the soul, which he called the animus, to become whole, it had to join with the anima, or the feminine aspect of the soul. The same is true of the feminine soul; the anima needs to join with its masculine aspect, the animus. When this happens, Jung claimed, the soul achieves balance and health, which he called individuation, the stated goal of Jungian psychotherapy or analysis.

In Integral Recovery, we must be aware of these two fundamental types. A masculine-identified individual will have different needs than a feminine-identified individual. One of the critiques of Alcoholics Anonymous, and one I feel is justified to some extent, is that successful white males designed AA.[1] This is seen clearly in AA's Twelve Steps; almost every step in some way involves ego deflation, which is a great need for the ego-inflated masculine alcoholic. If, however, we are treating a crack-addicted prostitute from the streets, there will probably be very little ego left intact, and what is left certainly does not need to be deflated, but supported and held in compassion. Using this perspective, we become more sensitive to our clients' developmental needs, instead of falling into the aforementioned cookie-cutter mode of treatment. This is the great advantage that a working knowledge of types gives us: it keeps us from being insensitive to the differences in individuals and helps us to be more compassionate and skillful.

In chapter 1, when we discussed the causative factors of chronic stress that lead directly to addiction, we referred to a lack of purpose, meaning, or connection in one's life. Masculine and feminine dimensions of addiction and the recovery process relate directly to this issue. For a masculine individual, it is crucial to rediscover a sense of purpose in life, to have a mission in the world, to be able to give one's unique gifts to the kosmos. Some higher meaning or value must become more important than the immediate gratification that comes from using drugs or alcohol, whether it is art, a meaningful career, or serving others. For a feminine individual, a greater meaning or value must also be discovered, but this time it will be interpreted in relational terms—loving others, being there for them, connecting in open-hearted communion. Both males and females need purpose and connection, but different individuals will emphasize one or the other, based on their type.[2] In any event, it is essential for a recovering individual to work on restoring both masculine purpose and feminine communion.

There are also specific masculine and feminine pathologies that must be resolved if they are present in a recovering individual. The pathological feminine will tend to lose her sense of self and overfocus on relationships, while the pathological masculine will tend toward narcissism and neglect of others and relationships. These tendencies are often exacerbated in the lives of middle- to late-stage addicts and need to be brought back into healthy balance or they will be a source of continuous disequilibrium, stress, and hence relapse.

Another useful way to view the masculine-feminine polarity is that addictive substances can be seen as the seduction of the negative feminine. You don't have to suffer. You don't have to feel pain. You don't have to face whatever you don't want to. I'll take away the pain. As with Odysseus' sirens, your life ends up shipwrecked on the rocks if you heed the sirens' song. Men and women truly lose their souls to this dark seduction; their life purpose and deepest relationships are forsaken. In later-stage addicts, we often see a vacuity in the eyes, the windows of the soul, or what was called by G.I.s in Vietnam, "the thousand-yard stare." Thus, the recovery process can also be seen as soul recovery. For the feminine soul, drugs can appear as the ultimate seduction of the negative masculine, offering domination, control, and protection from the vagaries and uncertainties of life, if one only yields one's personal autonomy and will.

A Brief Overview of the Enneagram

The Enneagram, I believe, is especially useful for Integral Recovery, as its primary purpose for centuries has been facilitating spiritual growth. In fact, I'm convinced that a whole book needs to be written on addiction

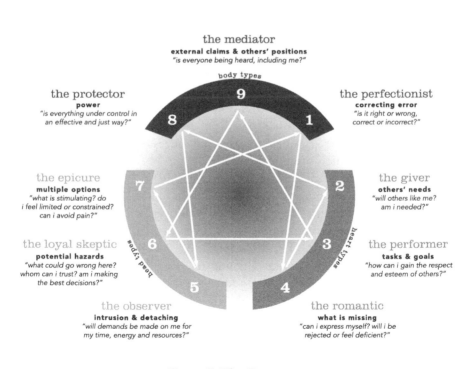

Figure 7. The Enneagram

Designed by Leigha Schneider

and the Enneagram, as I think that certain types are attracted to particular drugs and drug-taking strategies. Depending on the type, the addictive trance can play to each individual's deepest needs and weaknesses. For now, I will include the following overview of the Enneagram and describe how we can use it as part of our Integral treatment of addiction.[3]

Type One: The Perfectionist

At their best, Ones are "dependable, reliable, honest, hard-working, fair, self-disciplined, wise, scrupulous, full of integrity, and idealistic." Ones, at their worst, are "critical, judgmental, inflexible, controlling, jealous, worriers, serious, obsessive, dogmatic, and righteous." The dominant passion for Ones is anger; a repeating habit is resentment; the higher mind aspect is said to be perfection; and the positive virtue that healthy Ones embody at their best is serenity. In treating a newly arrived One, we might expect to see many of their negative qualities during their initial time in treatment.

As treatment progresses, we would expect to see their positive qualities emerge. One of the things that has most amazed me, and continues to be a source of wonder, is to watch students rapidly move from their Mr. Hyde negative aspects to their Dr. Jekyll healthy self. Considering the One's passion of anger and repeating habit of resentment, we would have strong indications of the issues that would have to be dealt with in treatment and some of the emotional problems that led the One to use drugs in the first place. Often, for example, a One's harsh judgment of others starts with deep self-judgment and self-condemnation. When Ones learn to accept and ultimately forgive themselves, this begins to cause a shift in their outward relations, and their sometimes unmerciful judgment becomes a more compassionate and skillful discrimination. I often see a softening in my One students, as compassion for self is mirrored in a growing compassion and acceptance of others, and more abiding peace, joy, and warm laughter begin to emerge.

Type Two: The Giver

Twos, at their best, are "empathetic, warm, supportive, appropriately generous, intuitive, adaptable, loving, loyal, selfless, and enthusiastic." Twos, at their worst, are "manipulative, smothering, gushing, possessive, give to get, indirect, hysterical, superior/aloof, seductive, and resentful." Twos' dominant passion is pride, and their repeating habit is flattery. Their higher mind manifests freedom, and the virtue most strongly manifested by the healthy Two is humility. Again, we would expect to see more of the negative qualities during the first few weeks of treatment. In an unhealthy Two client, we often find not only an addiction to drugs, but an addiction to people, or codependency. In other words, Twos give themselves away in an unhealthy attempt to control others. Very often, this is clearly what led to the original wounding and drug usage in the first place. So, for our clinicians and Integral Recovery team, as well as our type Two students themselves, this gives us a promising direction to explore, uncover, identify, release, and heal. Twos must look at this dual addiction: one to drugs, and one to people. Again, as our students begin to move their locus of control from their addict self to their healthy self, we would expect to see the healthy qualities of Twos emerge, which gives us points of strength to work with on the journey of recovery.

Type Three: The Performer

Threes, at their best, are "enthusiastic, adaptable, generous motivators, decisive, authentic, practical, optimistic, confident, industrious, and self-motivated." At their worst, they are "vain, narcissistic, overly competitive, deceptive, pretentious, ruthless, impatient, superficial, emotionally unavailable, and acquisitive." The Three passion is deceit; the repeating habit is vanity; the higher mind aspect is hope; and the positive virtue powerfully manifested by the healthy type Three is honesty. So we would expect to see, in our newly arrived Three student, a great deal of denial and justification regarding her drug use and subsequent behaviors. The good news with Threes is that once they commit to an Integral program of recovery and transformation, they will do it with the skill and motivation that they apply to almost every other task in their lives, including, unfortunately, getting and taking drugs. We would expect the Three in our group to become a good role model for other students in discipline, motivation, and enthusiasm. Good stuff, indeed!

Type Four: The Romantic

Fours, at their best, are "artistic, empathetic, creative, outgoing, warm, supportive, helpful, compassionate, intuitive, and expressive." At their worst, they are "over-dramatic, self-absorbed, moody, obsessively jealous, depressed, guilt-ridden, intractable, withdrawn, moralizing, shame-ridden, and rejecting." The Four passion is envy; repeating habit is melancholy; higher mind is connection with original essence; and the great virtue of the healthy type Four is equanimity. Fours, as our tragic-romantic poets, have no problem traveling into their interiors; however, they tend to get lost in them. Often, we think we have done great work when we get a Four in touch with his emotions, but this is actually no big deal for a Four. Getting lost in their emotions is where Fours may start having problems. For them to organize their interiors and bring forth their sensitivity, intelligence, and creativity, they need to find a purpose or a cause outside of themselves that helps them do this inner healing and self-organizing. Without this, our dear Fours fall into self-absorbed depression and angst. A healthy Four, however, is a true joy to be around and behold. There is a depth, sensitivity, and creativity that is rarely matched by any other type.

Type Five: The Observer

Fives, at their best, are "sensitive, wise, objective, have integrity, self-contained, perceptive, thoughtful, calm in a crisis, and loyal." At their worst, they are "arrogant, mean, emotionally unavailable, critical of others, negative, stubborn, reclusive, distant, and detached." Their passion is avarice, the fear being there is never enough to go around, especially never enough "me"; their repeating habit is stinginess; their higher mind is omniscience; and their virtue is nonattachment. One of the qualities that we find in an unhealthy Five is that they appear to be dead from the neck down; they live in their heads. In healing the Five, we must open up other areas such as the heart, the emotional life, and so forth—basically reconnecting the heart with the mind. As our Five students heal, their natural intelligence emerges, and often they fall into the role of the wise counselor within their peer groups, where they are consequently looked upon with respect because of their intelligence and wisdom. For the Integral Recovery team and therapist, a lot of work done with type Five students will center on dealing with their emotionally dissociative aspect—the split between intellect and feelings.

Type Six: The Questioner

Sixes, at their best, are "compassionate, warm, dutiful, reliable, hard working, practical, caring, witty, likeable, and loyal." At their worst, they are "paranoid, controlling, defensive, tetchy, unpredictable, judgmental, rigid, sarcastic, rebellious, and insecure." The Six passion is doubt; the repeating

habit is cowardice; the higher mind is faith; and the strong virtue of the
healthy Six is courage. Sixes are interesting because there are two pre-
dominating types: the first is a paranoid or phobic Six type. This would
be your "the sky is falling," scared-of-their-own-shadow type. The other
type is the counter-phobic Six, who appears to be very brave indeed,
doing many things that proves her courage and lack of fear. For example,
martial arts classes and military special forces are full of Six types. But
whether one is reacting to fear or against fear, the basic issue is the same.
Because the basic issue is fear, we would expect that the original emotional problems, the ones that our type Six students were using drugs to
resolve, are centered around fear, which often manifests in anxiety and
depression. But when a Six becomes healthy and begins to commit to
his own Integral Recovery process, we would expect him to manifest
great courage and tenacity in his healing journey.

Type Seven: The Epicure

Sevens, at their best, are "optimistic, enthusiastic, curious, entrepreneurial,
imaginative, spontaneous, productive, fun loving, charming, and confident."
At their worst, they are "rebellious, narcissistic, scattered, uncommitted,
undisciplined, impulsive, self-destructive, manic, over-talkative, and insensitive." A Seven's passion is gluttony; her repeating habit is rationalizing; her
higher aspect is sobriety; and her virtue is constancy. A Seven will often
behave like a honeybee going from flower to flower, collecting all the
nectar from life that she can. The problem with this is that an unhealthy
Seven becomes shallow. A Seven personality normally represents a certain
strategic response to early wounding (this is not to say that Sevens are
the only types that are formed around early wounding), and her particular
strategy of pleasure seeking is going from one thing to another, in an
effort to avoid that painful wound. As you might suspect, the direction
of healing for the Seven is to identify, feel, and release their shadow or
repressed aspect. When they do this inner healing shadow work, they are
remarkable creatures and are a joy to be around. Instead of shallowness,
healthy Sevens have a rather unique ability to see the depth of the beauty
in the world and to share that with others.

Type Eight: The Boss

Eights, at their best, are "protective, loyal, energetic, authoritative, honest,
fair, persistent, direct, straightforward, unpretentious, and self-confident."

At their worst, they are "bombastic, controlling, aggressive, insensitive, rebellious, antiauthoritarian, self-centered, domineering, skeptical, contentious, and ruthless." The passion of an Eight is lust; the repeating habit is vengeance; their higher aspect is truth; and the healthy Eight virtue is innocence. Working with them in recovery is often remarkable because of their capacity and tendency to cut through the bullshit and get to the heart of the matter. For more sensitive souls, this can be very frightening. But for those interested in truth, it can be exhilarating. An unhealthy Eight, on the other hand, is likely to be quite sociopathic in their inability to be empathetic toward others. However, the healthy Eight can be marvels to behold as the positive qualities above suggest. They can be amazing leaders and just the kind of people you would want to have "your back."

Type Nine: The Mediator

Nines, at their best, are "excellent mediators, reassuring, non-judgmental, patient, peaceful, receptive, empathetic, generous, gentle, and pleasant." At their worst, they are "stubborn, obsessive, passive-aggressive, spaced out, non-assertive, absent-minded, apathetic, judgmental, forgetful, and overly accommodating." The Nine passion is sloth; repeating habit is indolence; higher aspect is love; and virtue is right action. As you might have already guessed, Nines are sensitive souls. This often means that they have rather porous personal boundaries, and when they are involved in group work, for example, they often have a hard time differentiating between their feelings and the feelings of others. Because they are so sensitive, the motivation for their original drug usage is often tied into trying to numb powerful feelings that are overwhelming to them. As sloth, or laziness, is one of the qualities of the unhealthy Nine, we might expect that our type Nine students would need more encouragement and more push to engage in their Integral Recovery Practices than other types. However, we shouldn't push too hard, because with a Nine a little push goes a long way.

So as you can see, there is much material to be explored here, and much wisdom, compassion, and skillfulness to be gained by understanding the different personality types. There are many more subtleties to the Enneagram system that I have not covered here, and I would encourage anyone interested in Integral Recovery to explore the Enneagram more deeply on the internet and in many of the excellent books that have been written on this subject.[4] By adding the types lens that the AQAL map provides for us, I believe that Integral Recovery will prove to be more skillful, efficient, and effective than prior treatment models that have neglected this very important, if not essential, aspect of the human personality.

7

Bringing It All Together

Integral Recovery Treatment

Body, mind, heart, soul, and spirit. Emotion and shadow. Masculine, feminine, types. All four quadrants. All available levels. All essential lines. States. All essential practices. Finally, it seems, all the pieces are in place to make the leap to an Integral approach to addiction recovery. My belief is that by integrating the following practices and making this a lifelong endeavor oriented toward optimal health and well-being as well as sobriety, all the essential bases in the hard work of addiction recovery are covered:

- body practices (strength training, aerobics, yoga, diet, supplements);

- mind practices (the AQAL framework, understanding addiction, lifelong learning);

- spirit practices (daily BWE meditation, soul recovery, contemplative prayer);

- shadow/emotion practices (therapy, releasing emotions, shadow and trauma work).

The metapractice that helps foster growth in all of these areas, to a great extent, is our daily BWE meditation practice.

After six years of religiously doing my own Integral Recovery Practice, I have realized how simple the process actually is. Four things cover the essentials: diet, exercise, meditation, and lifelong learning. At the beginning of Integral Recovery treatment, the practice will be more intense, because treatment providers will give clients a big shove to get a healthy momentum going in their lives, to rebalance and rebuild their exhausted brains, bodies, minds, and spirits. Let's look more closely at how Integral Recovery treatment works in practice.

Integral Recovery begins with an Integral assessment of all quadrants, lines, levels, and types. Where does our client stand in the physical, cognitive, spiritual, emotional, and ethical aspects at his or her current stage of development? An initial Integral assessment might include the following:

- a thorough physical and nutritional evaluation (to include an evaluation of the medications that an individual has used in the past or is currently taking), assessing the overall state of physical fitness and the damage that has already been done through the abuse of a particular substance or substances;

- a detailed and up-to-date history of the individual's drug use;

- a psychosocial assessment of current life stressors, mental health issues, relationship issues, and psychological status;

- a family assessment, to examine particular nurturing and limiting functions of this key support system;

- an assessment of the developmental moral/value stage prior to the onset of the addictive process and the current stage center of gravity;

- a motivational interviewing[1] process, guided by the client's primary therapist, to access intrinsic motivation and help the client identify and overcome resistances to treatment. This process specifically helps the client with her resistances to growth and healing, i.e., asking, What is good about using? What are some of the negatives? What are the negatives about being here? What are some of the good things that could come from this experience?

- a spiritual evaluation to determine current beliefs, present and prior religious affiliations, and spiritual experiences and practices;

- an evaluation of the basic lines of intelligence, from which a current psychograph can be developed and studied in the context of developing an IRP that is optimal for the client's current needs. For example, an NFL running back who is addicted to pain medication would not start with the same physical exercise regimen as a couch-potato alcoholic;

- an all-quadrant evaluation that considers the client's resources: personal, financial, family, religious, community support, etc.;

- an assessment of outstanding cultural issues and how they might affect the treatment process, as in the difference between how an alcoholic is viewed in the Irish Catholic culture, where the drunk is often seen as a divine fool or poet, as opposed to in the Mormon culture, where drinking alcohol is strictly verboten.

At the end of the client's initial evaluation, and especially after the first week or so of working together, both Integral treatment provider and client will have a very clear understanding of:

- the work that must be done in all four quadrants;

- the work that must be done in all essential lines;

- the current moral stage of development;

- the moral stage of development the client was at before the onset of the disease;

- the causative factors that got the individual using in the first place, which need to be worked on in order for recovery to be complete and lasting;

- an understanding of the basic type of the individual, which is a huge help both in expanding the client's self-understanding and in informing the treatment team of the individual's needs and egoic inclinations.

As stated elsewhere in the book, this allows us to get away from a cookie-cutter approach to treatment, becoming more nuanced, subtle, and therefore effective in treating individuals. Then, as the client begins to understand the AQAL model and integrate it as an operating system, during the early weeks of treatment, we have a valuable, new, and very useful language that covers the whole journey of recovery in its many dimensions. I cannot stress how great a breakthrough it is having this map to use as a guide and tool in the recovery process.

Here, I will outline the sequence of treatment in an Integral Recovery program, describing the responsibilities of the treatment provider.

1. First, initiate the client into the program and make him feel welcome. Beginning treatment can be a scary and traumatic experience for the newly arrived. There may be great fear around stopping the relationship with the addictive substance(s), since obtaining and taking the particular drug(s) has become the center of the addicted person's life. Questions arise such as, Can I do this? Will I always feel as bad as I do right now? Who are these people? Can they help me? Do I really want or need help?

2. Work with an attitude of receptivity, compassion, and respect, each of which is very important in helping the client become enrolled in his or her own recovery process. Massage/bodywork, reiki, saunas, or sweats can be of great assistance in this regard, through establishing the belief that recovery involves a relief from suffering.

3. Quickly initiate a regimen of nutritional recovery, which includes the appropriate supplements (vitamins, amino acids, minerals, herbs, and essential fatty acids) to counteract the pathological effects of drugs and alcohol on the body and brain, as well as improving the diet.

4. Teach a series of introductory classes, using multimedia, to explain the Integral Recovery model, to include the AQAL map and the neuroscience behind the disease of addiction.

5. Define an appropriate Integral physical workout practice, including stretching (yoga), strength training, and aerobic exercise.

6. Enlighten the client about the many contemplative/spiritual practices available and initiate BWE meditation. This style of meditation may be the "missing link" in the recovery world, as it produces rapid results by putting practitioners in states of deep meditation right from the start, without years of prior

training and practice. For addicts, waiting for years is not a viable option.[2]

This technology seems to facilitate healing and relief from trauma and deep-seated depression, often primary causes of chronic relapse for the addict. The data[3] indicates that in the deep theta or delta states of meditation, formerly split-off, repressed material comes into awareness and, with the appropriate therapeutic meditation techniques, can be accepted, integrated, and released. Healing from trauma is a key component of an Integral Recovery approach. One study indicates that fully 60 percent of women alcoholics suffered sexual abuse as children.[4] As mentioned before, in Dan Siegel's work on using mindfulness and meditation to treat mental illness,[5] he states that mental illness is characterized by rigidity and chaos, while mental health is characterized by coherence and integration. The meditative practices and shadow work of IR quickly begin to lead the student away from this pathological rigidity and chaos to more coherence and integration, both in the Upper-Right functioning of the brain and the Upper-Left release and transmutation of the split off and shadow elements in the psyche.

7. Use the above-mentioned BWE technologies coupled with recorded affirmations,[6] another very promising healing modality based on the pioneering work of Michael Murphy, George Leonard, and others.[7]

8. Continue individual therapy and group therapy, as in traditional treatment, but with a great deal more energy and efficacy, as the synergistic effects of the other Integral Recovery Practices deepen the level of participation and engagement.

9. After each meditation period, give the client time to journal his experiences, and follow this with a process group. These groups, affected by the therapeutic inroads made possible by the BWE-enhanced meditation, are more effective and occur at a deeper and more real level than groups we held prior to using this type of meditation practice.

Wilderness as a context and part of an Integral Recovery program is another option. Research sponsored by the Outdoor Behavioral Healthcare

Industry Council (OBHIC)[8] has shown that bonded, trusting relationships happen more rapidly and at a deeper level in the wilderness milieu
than in any other traditional residential treatment modality. In addiction
treatment, this bonded, trusting relationship is essential in creating the
precondition for growth and healing to happen. We have found that in
Integral Recovery treatment, because we meditate and practice together,
these close emotional bonds are also quickly established.

Other benefits of a wilderness setting include learning humility before the grandeur and impartiality of nature, working together
with others, and a host of other lessons that facilitate the move from
pathological egocentrism to a more caring response for self and others.
The potential for spiritual awakening is also greatly enhanced during
prolonged forays into the wilderness. Baker Roshi[9] is quoted as saying,
"Enlightenment is an accident, but meditation makes one more accident
prone." For years, I have watched clients become more "accident prone"
sleeping under the stars, sitting around the fire, and journeying through
the canyons, mountains, and deserts.

Vision Questing

I have used vision quests for many years now. I started out vision questing myself and, later, used vision quests as one of the major interventions
in the Passages to Recovery (PTR) program. At PTR, we would begin
preparing students for their vision quests the very first week. We would
find, almost across the board, that students were enthusiastic about partici-
pating in a vision quest, from having seen and heard about the results of
the senior students who had already done theirs. In my Integral Recovery work, which has been largely conducted in Wayne County, Utah, an
amazing wilderness area, I would estimate that at least 50 percent of my
students have chosen vision questing as an option in their healing and
deepening process.

What is a vision quest? A vision quest is based on ancient Native
American rite of passage ceremonies, most often done by boys making the
transition to adulthood and sometimes by women in training to become
healers or shamans. There are similar practices in cultures around the
world. This can be seen in the Bible, and perhaps most dramatically in
Jesus' life in the Gospels, when he goes away to pray in solitude. During
his 40 days in the wilderness, he is confronted by the devil, or perhaps

his own demons, the victory over which initiates him and prepares him to start his teaching ministry.

In the current Integral Recovery program, our vision quests, sometimes called Prayer Fasts, are conducted at a forechosen spot, or a sacred place. I often tell students to find a place where it would be good to die, as symbolically what is occurring on the vision quest is the death and burying of the old addict way of life and the birth of the new, sober, purposeful, and ethical life. When a student has decided on her spot, we come back a few days later to do an initial inquiry process, in which I help her find the purpose of her vision quest.

The question that I always have students ask and ponder is, What am I going to make so? In modern times, vision quests are often used to mark life transitions, such as going from being single to being married, from being married to being a parent, from being a student to moving into one's career, to mark a divorce or retirement from a prior life's work, and so on. In the case of my students, vision quests deal largely with their recovery and sobriety issues. When the students have ascertained the purpose of their quest, I instruct them that they are out there foremostly to pray, to empty themselves, and to seek divine strength, healing, and direction for their lives. As it says quite beautifully in the Eleventh Step of Alcoholics Anonymous, "Sought through prayer and meditation to improve our conscious contact with God as we understood him, praying only for the knowledge of his will for us and the power to carry that out." This is a beautiful summary of the purpose of the vision quest.

Often my students build a sacred circle, or circle of intention, in which they stay during the vision quest (except to use the facilities, as it were). They then divide the circle into the four quadrants and spend time praying and meditating in each quadrant, seeking both divine help and understanding of the work that must be done in each quadrant on their journey of healing and recovery. I allow them to take a journal with them to record their experience and insights. This seems to help deepen the process.

More recently, I have also allowed my students to take their iPods or CDs, with only their meditation tracks, to help them in their meditative and contemplative work. When I first considered this, I ran into resistance in my own mind, thinking, well, that's certainly not traditional. But, then I asked myself, what tradition exactly are you upholding here? And the answer was, none. Since then, I have repeatedly found that this 21st-century addition to the vision quest works incredibly well.

The vision quest is not for everyone. But for those who make the decision to do it, I have found it extremely useful. When one moves into one's sacred vision quest space, whatever occurs there is a part of a mythical and sacred journey. Even when students occasionally choose not to complete their quests, there is a powerful lesson to be learned and interpreted. In other words, with insightful and wise mentoring, even apparent failures can become successes and opportunities to learn and grow.

The end of a student's quest is followed by a sacred meal that is healthy and easily digestible for one who has been fasting for three days— usually a vegetable soup of some sort—followed by a council, in which the student shares her experience or vision and is aided by a guide in interpreting and putting her vision into the context of her life. I often teach that a vision quest begins when one decides to go on the quest, and that the most difficult and, indeed, important part of the quest is not the time alone and fasting itself, but living the wisdom and guidance that one has been shown on the mountain or in the sacred place. As a native elder once said, upon hearing a grandiose vision from someone who had come off a quest, "But will it grow corn?" In other words, the purpose of the vision quest is not just to achieve altered states, but to achieve inner transformation and altered traits and behaviors, as well as direction, and to bring this back into the world, thereby blessing one's people and relationships. In the Lakota language, the most common greeting is, "*Metaquiescen*," which means "all our relations," a wonderful teaching in itself. Whatever we do affects all our relations, and in determining our life, our goals, and our practices, we must always include this knowledge that it is not only about us but about all our relations.

Family

Another important aspect of the Integral Recovery program is family involvement. Family systems theory has long recognized that individual pathologies do not happen in a vacuum but are created and flourish in the "intersubjective" dimension, the Lower-Left quadrant. It is understood that addiction is a family syndrome, with different individuals playing their part in the dance: the addict, the enabler, the martyr, and so forth. The job of Integral treatment is to treat not just the "identified patient" but the whole family. Part of this approach with family means that an

Integral Recovery Practice is prescribed for everyone. Everyone becomes involved in his or her own practice and awakening process, as is age, type, and stage appropriate. This creates movement, change, and often some chaos, which facilitates the whole system to move to a higher state of functioning.

Healthy Communication

Integral Recovery clients must learn the basics of honest communication and reflective listening. Often we feel that good communication consists of winning the argument. As a pretty darn good arguer myself, I can assure you that this is not the case, unless you are on a debating team. What matters in healthy communication is that we express our thoughts and feelings honestly, that we are heard, and at the same time that we deeply hear those whom we are in dialogue with.

One of the skills that I've incorporated and used over the years in working with addicts and their families is called motivational interviewing (MI).[10] MI is a practice that helps our clients come to their own truth, recognize where they are in their lives, and develop a motivation for change that comes from within. The underlying assumption is that the truth that comes from *your* mouth about you is more powerful than the truth that comes from my mouth about you. In the early stages of treating addiction, when there is great denial and resistance to the idea that there might be a problem and you might have to change your way of doing things, this is incredibly useful. The practice of MI is quite complex, but I believe that I have boiled it down to its bare essentials, which can be taught and learned rather easily with practice.

Here is an example of how it works. If a client emphatically and passionately cries, "I don't want to be here!" then one does not say, "But you need to be here, because . . ." Instead one reflects back, with the same passion and intensity, "You really don't want to be here!" Immediately, the person feels heard and resistance begins to diminish. And the conversation continues, "My mother is a bitch. She's the one who needs to be here!" Then I reflect back with passion, "So, your mother is a bitch, and you think she needs to be here too!" He responds, "Yeah. And it's not fair." And I respond back, "And you really think it's not fair." And he responds, "Yes." At this point, the intensity begins to deescalate, and the conversation deepens. Then the student might say something like,

"My god, my life is such a mess." And I can then respond in a gentler tone, "Yes, it's hard."

At this point, the client feels heard, respected, and emotionally connected with me, although I'm not necessarily agreeing with anything he just said. Now I might sit next to him, as opposed to across from him, and perhaps suggest something like, "Do you want to look at this? Let's look at what really sucks about being in treatment." He will spark up at this and may respond with things like, "I miss my girlfriend. I have no freedom. My parents lied to me, etc." After I reflect back to him all the things that suck about being in treatment, I will repeat them back as a list, and then say, "Have I got it right?" He may respond with, "Yes," or, "No, you missed something." Then we complete that portion of the interview. Then I can ask the question, "On the other hand, what are maybe some of the good things that could come from your being here?" He may say something like, "Maybe I can get healthy again." Or, "I could earn back some of the trust that I have lost with my parents." "Maybe there are a few things I could learn here about being sober." I then reflect back all the possible positive things there could be about treatment for this client, and again go back over the negative things there are about being here. Then I'll say, "Given all the bad things about being here, and given the positive things that could come from being here, where are you on a scale of one to ten? One being I can't handle this; I've gotta run right now. And ten being I am completely done with drugs, and I need to be here to get and stay sober. The client will usually say, "Maybe a four or a five (or some other number)." And I'll say, "Great; good job."

At this point, we have deescalated the conflict and the client has been able to step back and view his predicament objectively, weighing the negatives and the positives. We have also been very respectful of where he is in his development process, and at the same time, have strengthened the connection between counselor and client. This is a very useful and powerful tool to use whenever there is ambivalence about any decision that needs to be made.

I often use this technique when looking at the client's drug use itself. I'll say something like, "Okay, let's look at your drug use. And let's look at what's really *good* about using drugs." At this point, if the client can see that I honestly want to know what she has to say about this and understands that I'm not asking in a manipulative or cynical way, she usually shows up enthusiastically and talks about all the great things about using drugs. For example, "It feels great! I love the taste! I have new friends. I like buying drugs! I love selling drugs!" At that point, I reflect back to her the good things, in her opinion, about using drugs. I say, "So, using drugs makes you feel great . . ."

After this discussion, I say, "Okay, good job. Now let's look at some of the things that may *not* be so good about using drugs." At this point, she is in the flow and feeling some trust toward me and is almost always ready to look at the negative aspects of her drug use. It might go like this: "Well, it's certainly screwing up my family relations . . . and my finances . . . and my education. And, sometimes, the hangovers or withdrawal symptoms are really terrible." Then at that point, I say, "Okay, so on the good side (and I hold up one hand as if I am weighing the issues), we have the good parts, drugs feel great, etc. And on the other hand, the negative parts are loss of respect from my family, educational failure, and so on." And again, having looked at both sides, both the negatives and the positives of using drugs, I ask, "Where do you feel you are right now, on a scale of one to ten, in your motivation to change and stop using drugs?" One being, no way do I want to change, I just want to use more drugs, and ten being, I'm here 100 percent, and I can never use again. Usually, they will come out as a 5 or 6 in their motivation, which I affirm and say, "Great job." After this, they will often ask, "Well, how long do I have to be here?" And I will say, "Well, how long do you think you need to be here?" and so on.

This is a very quick way of building rapport and trust and really gets us over the idea that counseling consists of winning the argument. It also allows them to understand their own motivation for change and the necessity for that change through their own eyes and their own mouths. It really is a brilliant practice, and I recommend it to all types of health care providers and to anyone seeking to improve their communication skills and the quality of their relationships. For example, in my personal life, I have learned that when my strong-willed wife and I begin to argue, and I don't feel like arguing, I can simply use the skills that I have developed working with MI to diffuse the situation. If my wife says something like, "I feel really disrespected when you don't wash the dishes," instead of replying, "My not washing the damn dishes has nothing to do with my respect for you one way or the other!" (at which point, the conversation would escalate dramatically in a negative direction), I can say, clearly and emphatically, matching her tone, "Honey, I hear you really feel disrespected when I don't wash the dishes." It is amazing how quickly the situation diffuses and harmony is restored. (Then I wash the dishes after enough time has passed that I can maintain some dignity.)

MI also works the opposite way. For example, if I am really angry and feeling very passionate and emphatic about something, and my wife feels threatened, I will say to her, "Honey, you had better MI me." And when she does, the winds of my passion abate quite quickly, and I feel heard. Again, harmony is restored.

This is a great technique that allows treatment and life to flow more skillfully and beautifully while wasting less time on confrontation and allowing for much more enjoyment of the process. Having said that, this does not mean that there are never times when one should be didactic and directive. But these moments are a lot more effective when a trusting relationship has been established, which is exactly what MI helps to do.

Developing such skills is very effective for a treatment provider, a husband or wife, a parent, or in our day-to-day interactions with others. For example, I was outside a store in a parking lot one summer and noticed that a child was locked in a car. I quickly enlisted other people in the vicinity to help me try to find the mother or father and then forced the car door open. We removed the toddler and a freaked-out, upset mother quickly arrived on the scene. She was very confused and ashamed and called her husband. The husband arrived on a large Harley Davidson motorcycle. He was a rough-looking character. He quickly got into it with me with a great deal of anger, and it looked as if I was going to have to physically defend myself. At that point, I kicked into MI mode and very quickly had the situation diffused and the husband thanking me.

One last note on this subject. Motivational interviewing works much better when there is actual caring and compassion behind the technique. The client will sense either caring or the lack of caring. In my experience, the old "You can't bullshit a bullshitter" saw holds true with most addicts. They can sense quite accurately whether you are being real or not.

Learning the motivational interviewing type of communication allows us to repair our relationships in the Lower-Left quadrant (the "we" quadrant of the IR model). Without attention to and skill in the Lower-Left quadrant, the harm done to the healing milieu as well as personal relationships will be a source of constant and toxic stress.

In the chapters to come, we will look at and examine in more detail the essential practices involved in the Integral Recovery model—practices intended to heal and balance the body, brain, heart, and soul.

8

Building the Body

Instead of a bar bill, pick up a barbell!

—John Dupuy

Ahhh, the body—the miraculous human body. It is our home, our temple, and the vehicle through which we experience our lives and give our gifts. In Integral Recovery, if the body is not restored, honored, and built to a high degree of optimal conditioning and health, recovery is not happening. Each individual with whom I have worked, addiction issues or not, who has gotten into the gym and made rigorous exercise a regular part of their lives has increased their health and happiness and made me look like a genius. Exercise and nutrition are not the whole story in the Integral approach, but they are a very big part, a foundational part. In this chapter, I will first discuss building the body with exercise and strength training and then I will explore building the body with proper food and supplementation—an essential part of our detoxification base camp and regeneration process.

It bears repeating here that one of the main principles of Integral Recovery is that good work done in any of the quadrants helps to lift up and heal each of the other quadrants. A strong healthy body will help you do healing and growth work in your interiors (Upper-Left quadrant); it will lend strength and support in the work on your relationships (Lower-Left quadrant); and it will support your overall successful interactions with and contributions to the world (Lower-Right quadrant). Other benefits include rolling back the biological clock, restoring healthy brain chemistry, alleviating and releasing stress, and replacing despair with a sense of health and well-being. You look better, you feel better; you just can't beat it. Here, again, are the words of a Quaker elder whom I remember reading years ago. "The key to lifelong happiness is to be a lifelong athlete."

My own strength-building practice is absolutely embedded in me; it is just what I do. And I do it with passion. I have had over a quarter century love affair with gyms and working out. When I am traveling and on the road, finding places to work out has the same importance as food, gas, and lodging. At fifty-five, I am physically stronger than I have ever been. I can bench press over three hundred pounds and don't think I have reached my upper limit yet. As Dominic Juliano says (a master and early pioneer of body building who works out at my gym), "Your muscles have no idea how old you are." Dominic must be somewhere in his seventies, and he is a specimen: energetic, vital, and strong as an ox.

It should come as no surprise that attaining physical health and well-being is the foundation of a successful recovery as well as a key to success and happiness. Starting from a place of ill health, this may seem daunting at first, but what you need to do is just get started. Remember, you are exercising for your life. You'll need help, support, and training to get going, but in short order, the good feelings that are generated from the healthy brain chemicals that exercise is releasing in your brain, along with seeing the positive results of your early practice, will make you actually look forward to your workouts. As a result of the positive changes that you experience, hope is reborn in your life. "If I can do this, feel, and be so much better, what can't I do?" As your hope, courage, and strength build in the gym, you begin to truly understand that the key to your recovery, health, and happiness is your discipline and dedication to your Integral Recovery Practice. There is a sign on the wall at a Gold's Gym I work out at in Salt Lake City that says, Know this: Commitment is a muscle, which is another way of saying that the more we commit to our commitment to practice, the easier it becomes and the stronger the commitment becomes.

One of the many serendipitous events that happened while writing this book was that while I was working on the first draft, Shawn Phillips' book *Strength for Life*[1] was published. Shawn is the brother of Bill Phillips, author of *Body for Life*,[2] a huge bestseller that has helped many people reach their hitherto unimagined fitness goals. Shawn was a partner in this process and helped his brother Bill develop a system and line of high-end supplements for over ten years.

What Shawn does in his book is give us twenty years of body-building and strength training experience, as well as a decade of working with his brother and the Fitness for Life program. He has evaluated why some people made it and some did not and added a spiritual dimension that he felt was missing in the bodybuilding world and, initially, in his own practice. What I think he has done is create a near-perfect fit for the physical line of the Integral Recovery model. What I don't intend to do here is regurgitate point by point what Shawn has written in his book, as he has already written it in a very concise and effective manner. But I would like to comment on how it applies to the goal of Integral Recovery.

First, Shawn defines health as synonymous with strength—not just the absence of disease. One could be the proverbial disease-free couch potato, living on Twinkies and soda pop, and in Shawn's world, and in our Integral Recovery world, this would not be called health by a long shot. When an addict begins Integral Recovery treatment, he is probably going to be very weak in all of his essential lines, and most likely, all four quadrants of his life will be a mess. By beginning with the body line, using the Strength for Life model that Shawn has developed, we will heal, strengthen, and optimize the very foundation of our lives—our body. Not only that, but our strength-training practice also restores health to our brain and helps us to recover our freedom, discipline, will power, and mastery of our lives.

Strength training causes the body to produce an array of chemicals on which the brain thrives. To name a few of the major ones, there are endorphins for a general sense of well-being; serotonin for mood regulation, sleep, and serenity; dopamine, which gives us the juice and joy to relish life; and epinephrine and norepinephrine, which give us energy and focus. Additionally, training stimulates the production of Brain-Derived Neurotropic Factor (BDNF) as well as Nerve Growth Factor (NGF), both of which are known to promote cell health and development in the brain, insulate the brain from the effects of both aging and stress, and facilitate high levels of "cognitive fitness," (i.e., help you to think clearly, make good decisions, and function with improved mental processing times).[3] All of this is a great help in reducing the stress that drives the overpowering cravings that are at the heart of the disease of addiction.

What Shawn recommends in his Strength for Life program is to begin with a 12-day period of detoxification, rest, renewal, light exercise, and stretching. This is exactly what we do in Integral Recovery. The first job is most certainly restoration, relaxation, and detoxification, so our clients begin to understand that sobriety and health feel a hell of a lot better than addiction and disease. As Shawn points out in his book, one of the main reasons that people who tried the Body for Life program did *not* succeed was that they were in a state of such stress and weakness before they hit the gym that the initial experience of exercise simply added more stress to their lives, causing them to give up their fitness goals.

After 12 days of regeneration and detoxification, fitness school starts with a 12-week intensive training program and a nutritional program that rebuilds and purifies the body as well as strengthening and healing the mind. This 12-week intensity, however, does not last throughout the year. As Shawn relates in his book, he was watching one of Lance Armstrong's amazing athletic performances in the Tour de France when he had a moment of deep insight. He realized that Lance was performing at such an incredible level, because he only trained for one race a year—namely, the Tour de France, the highlight of the bike-racing world. Lance did not train intending to stay at his peak condition all year long; rather, he trained to be at his peak condition at the exact time of the race.

This was a breakthrough moment for Shawn and a breakthrough moment for me as I read his book. As a result, Shawn recommends that we go through three or four training cycles a year, and after each 12-week program, we knock off for a week. By repeating this pattern of 12-week training periods followed by a week's downtime for simply relaxing, we keep growing and optimizing ourselves while keeping it interesting and challenging. I believe this is a brilliant model.

Shawn uses a pyramid to help explain his model. The primary focus of each cycle of training is represented by the apex of the pyramid. For example, during the first 12-week training cycle, the apex of the pyramid might be strength training. This means that during these 12 weeks, the main exercise is strength training, but the program also includes a secondary focus on both cardio and stretching, which are the bases of the pyramid. After the first training cycle and a week off, the practice at the apex (or top of the pyramid) will change, for example, to cardio, which is now the primary exercise, while still including strength training and stretching/yoga as the bases. During the third 12-week cycle, stretching/yoga would be the apex, and the program would also include a lesser focus on strength training and cardio. After this period, one would begin again with strength training at the top of the pyramid.

Shawn's model for strength training also includes something he calls Focus Intensity Training (FIT). This is a process of bringing absolute intentionality and focus to your strength training. This serves not only to give your training a depth of meaning, something it often lacks in popular strength training and body building culture, but it also trains and strengthens the mind in such a way that it will positively strengthen your recovery and the pursuit of your dreams and life goals. Anyone who has suffered from the disease of addiction, or knows someone who has, can clearly see that addiction is a destroyer of dreams, purpose, and meaning in the addict's life. As stated earlier, we are not just practicing our Strength for Life practices to look better and feel better; we are practicing for our very lives.

Integral Recovery training gives us a method of immediately creating peak states and positive moods and mental attitudes. I often go to the gym when I am mentally exhausted and physically tired, and as soon as I begin my intensely focused strength training, I experience a great sense of renewed strength, vitality, and mental clarity. This is a wonderful skill to cultivate, as we can learn to use our exercise as a substitute for unhealthy activities or using addictive substances.

The ability to create peak states, in which we are focused, calm, and confident, can be trained into an enduring trait that permeates well beyond the gym. I know that my strength training was a great aid to me when I approached the challenge of writing this book. The focus and the confidence I gained from the gym readily translated into focus and

What **focus intensity training** (FIT) does is enable us to focus completely, with total concentration, on the exercise at hand and even the specific muscle being exercised. This gives us, in addition to increased muscular strength, new mental abilities such as clarity and focus. Between exercises, we practice complete relaxation, which is an aspect of our muscular strength training and which has the added benefit of teaching us how to deal with stress in everyday life as it arises. Another key aspect of FIT lies in the visualization of our routine before we hit the gym. For example, in my case, I do this while I'm driving to the gym. Let me stipulate here that I live in a *very* unpopulated area, and I'm able to accomplish this without running into anybody (knock on wood). When I get to the gym, and before I begin my workout, I sit quietly for a few moments and dedicate my practice to the highest good that I can conceive of. This serves to give a depth of meaning and inspiration to the practice and helps strengthen the resolve to continue to practice.

courage when it came to writing what you are now reading. Strength training helps us to remain grounded in the face of obstacles—an aspect of the "training state" that you will soon know well. Touching into this state, this break from the many stresses of life outside of training can become a powerful respite from life, especially at times when life is experienced as hell (which happens); it's a tremendous help in preventing relapse. Strength training also creates a whole other domain for practicing awareness, in addition to our daily meditation. These two practices, meditation and strength training, work synergistically so that both practices become more powerful.

The true proof of the pudding is, in addition to providing a very pleasurable and effective means of achieving growth and sustained sobriety, the real wonder of how we feel even when we are not practicing. Strength and focus begin to diffuse throughout our whole life. "Trained state" experiences actually accumulate, which allows for higher stage growth. Both our meditation and strength training are creating greater horizontal health, which translates into happiness and effectiveness at our present stage of growth, while also enabling us to move expeditiously and efficiently to our next stage of development. We could say that, in addition to horizontal health and vertical growth, we will be experiencing greater "essential" health, which means that these practices will help us tap into our own essential nature and help us to realize who we really are in the deepest and most profound sense.

Here, I will quote Shawn at some length. What he is saying about the Strength for Life program is equally true, if not doubly true, as it applies to Integral Recovery because of the practice or die motivation that we bring to our IRP.

> The secret of reaching your potential is in the unlimited capacity of the body, mind, heart, and soul that can only be found deep within, where your true strength arises. Most people never know the true depth of their strength because they have never been tested or pushed to find out what they are made of—physically, mentally, spiritually. When you discover this unshakable belief in your strength, you begin to open to what you're here for and can do with this lifetime. Ultimately, the measure of your life is in the difference you can make in this world—in your impact on others. Doing more, being more, and giving more calls upon your reservoir of strength.

Only with considerable capacity can you be in a position to do the most for others and be of the greatest service to those who mean the most in your life.

Again, the challenge and adventure of Integral Recovery takes us to the deepest, strongest, and best part of ourselves. As an Integral Recovery student and practitioner, you are not just going to survive; you are going to transform yourself and the world around you.

The World of Integral Nutrition

I have said that nutrition is the foundation of Integral Recovery, and by that I mean that it supplies the first layer of groundwork, in the Upper Right quadrant, for our entire healing journey. Ken Wilber once said that nature is foundational to human civilization, because if human civilization were to disappear, could nature carry on? Absolutely! Not a problem. If nature were to disappear, however, could human civilization carry on? No how; no way. Put another way, if we destroyed all the molecules in the universe, there would still be plenty of atoms because atoms are foundational to molecules—just as nature is foundational to our human world. In the same way, nutrition is the foundation and the starting point of our Integral approach to recovery. For example, when I pick people up at the Salt Lake City airport to drive them south to work with me, the first thing I give them when they get into the car, besides a handshake and a hug, is a bottle full of pure water and a hand-ful of supplements. The message is: God bless you, brother or sister, your healing journey has begun.

As we have said before, addiction is a disease that affects the brain, and in the brain of the addict, there will be extreme depletion of essen-tial neurochemicals. This leads to imbalance and suffering in the life of the addict. With our supplementation and diet, we immediately begin the process of rebuilding the brain by supplying the nutritional building blocks that support our work. If optimal neurochemical balance is not restored, and if physical health is not restored, the stress and cravings that the addicted person will continue to suffer almost certainly assure relapse, time and again.

Here, I will outline a basic supplement regimen to get you started. First, I recommend a top-shelf, organic multivitamin that includes minerals as well as vitamins and is rich in fruits, vegetables, green foods, enzymes, amino acids, bioflavonoids, herbs, and essential fatty acids.[4] I also recommend oils that supply the omega-3, omega-6, and omega-9 fatty acids, which are essential for restoring healthy brain function and are very effective in combating depression, energy crashes, and the cravings associated with addiction. Your best bet in this department is probably using fish oils (krill oil is said to be very good). It is important to note that you should use pharmaceutical-grade fish oil so that all the impurities have been removed from the oil before you ingest it. Although pharmaceutical-grade oils are more expensive, you can use them without the risk of ingesting environmental toxins. Also, if you have problems with eating fish for vegetarian or spiritual reasons, I recommend Udo's Flaxseed Oil, especially the one that includes DHA, a powerful essential nutrient not normally found in vegetarian oils. In this case, it comes from green foods such as spirulina.

I also recommend supplementing with a high-grade multiamino acid supplement. There are many of these on the market. And another product I like to use is chlorella,[5] which is treated in such a way that its cellular walls are cracked, making it almost completely absorbable by the body. Besides being a great source of pure protein and green nutrients, chlorella has been shown to be very effective in detoxing the body from heavy metals and other pollutants.

The list goes on. I have found that kudzu capsules are helpful because they are antioxidants, and, interestingly, they have been used in Chinese medicine for centuries to decrease cravings for alcohol. I have seen very good results in the people I have worked with, and the testimonials of others have been equally positive. I also recommend a product called Super Enzymes,[6] which supports healthy digestion and aids in breaking down fats, carbohydrates, and proteins, while optimizing nutritional absorption. This may seem like a lot, and it *is* a lot, but, remember, you are playing "catch up." There is a lot of healing, balancing, and rebuilding work to be done.

There are many in-depth and very good books on detoxification and nutrition, which I will list at the end of this chapter, but let me offer a few basic principles of nutrition right here. Ultimately, each person has to find a nutritional plan that works for her, as we all have different nutritional needs and respond better to different diets, depending on our genetic makeup, gender, current age, and so on. But, across the board, I think I can safely say that there are certain things we need to avoid.

These are all of the highly processed foods: junk food, macaroni and cheese, fast foods, the sorts of things that assault you in convenience stores, white flour, processed sugar often disguised under the label of corn syrup, unhealthy fats, too much salt, and unhealthy carbohydrates. We also want to avoid toxic chemicals, preservatives, and other unhealthy substances. In fact, you will know that you are getting healthier when you enter a convenience store and feel almost ill just looking at its offerings. (In emergency situations, I go for unsalted roasted nuts or sunflower seeds and get the hell out of there. I have also learned to bring a cooler with good food for long road trips. It makes traveling much healthier and the time I save at fast food joints, I spend at the gym.)

Our basic guidelines should be "lean, clean, and green." Lean means going easy on fats and using healthy fats, such as flaxseed and olive oil, instead of trans fats. Organic nut oils are good too. As far as carbohydrates go, one should focus on whole grains, brown rice, and quinoa. Whole grain carbohydrates break down into sugar for energy as do all carbohydrates, but they break down more slowly than processed foods such as white flour, giving us sustained energy versus sugar-induced spikes that pick us up and then crash us down, with the resulting loss of energy and weight gain.

As far as clean goes, we want to go organic all the way, not only with the food we eat, but also with the products we use such as shampoo, soap, and housecleaning products. There is a great deal of ever-increasing evidence that environmental toxins lead to disease and destroy our health. In the case of addiction, this simply leads to further self-medication and drug use. When I say organic, I mean foods must be labeled organic according to the USDA. "All natural" does not necessarily mean organic, and labeling can be very deceptive. If you are lucky enough to live in a major urban area, you will find great organic grocery stores available. Not only do these stores have a good variety of supplements, but they also offer fresh, healthy meats, vegetables, and fruits. You pay a little more, but you get a lot more out of what you eat. I have also found that if you order your supplements online, you can save a great deal of money. All of this takes time and effort, but so did taking drugs. As I've said before, I often ask my students, "How much time did you spend obsessing about and taking drugs?" And almost inevitably, the answer will be, "24/7." So get with the program. It is fun and highly rewarding.

In order to be green, we should eat as many green vegetables and fruits as possible, and the more pigmentation (or deeper the color), the better. This goes for fruits and vegetables of all colors, but especially green ones. In *The Detox Revolution*, Thomas J. Slaga and Robin Kueneke tell us "all colorful fruits and vegetables, inside or out, contain flavonoids, carotenoids, or other beneficial phytochemicals with important anti-oxidant properties . . . The same phytochemicals that cause the color also inhibit inflammation; lower cholesterol; and prevent cancer, heart disease, and other illnesses. The phytochemical chlorophyllin, which is found in the pigment of green vegetables and fruits, has recently been established to have such abilities."[7]

To build on the wisdom of AA, which uses the acronym HALT (meaning avoid being hungry, angry, lonely, and tired), we should not let ourselves get hungry. Especially in early recovery, hunger pangs lead to cravings for alcohol, which turns to sugar in our blood streams. Therefore, we should eat more small, healthy meals a day versus a few very large meals. This keeps us from experiencing hunger and energy crashes and speeds up our metabolism, so we lose unwanted weight. This was a hard one for me, as in the last few years before my personal Integral practice revolution, I was eating one large meal a day. Now I'm up to four meals a day, five on a good day. I find protein shakes very tasty and satisfying,[8] and I like to have organic almonds and fruit in the kitchen to munch on between meals. I've noticed that my energy is a lot higher, and I feel better overall.

Many authors say that one day a week, we can perhaps indulge ourselves without causing too much harm. Could be; it's a nice thought, but I'm not sure if it is true. But, for example, if you are conscious about your diet throughout the year, enjoying a traditional American Thanksgiving meal with second and third helpings will probably not destroy your life, so you can relax on that score. Another thing I've learned is that eating well takes awareness and planning. Again, as stated earlier, if you are preparing to go on a trip either flying or driving, it is important to bring enough healthy food along with you to get you through the nutritional wastelands that we often travel through in the United States.

In the excellent and much recommended book *Integral Life Practice*,[9] the authors (Ken Wilber, Terry Patton, Adam Leonard, and Marco Morelli) break nutrition down into four quadrants. In the Upper-Left quadrant, they recommend we eat mindfully. This means with attention and awareness. If we practice eating mindfully, it becomes increasingly difficult to ingest foods that are unhealthy. In the Lower-Left quadrant, they suggest that we eat meaningfully in that we actually use our meals as opportunities to deepen our relationships and increase the spiritual quality of our lives. In the Lower-Right quadrant, they suggest we eat sustainably, becoming aware of the environmental impacts of our food choices, and therefore supporting local and organic growers and sustainable businesses that employ compassion and kindness to the animals that are used as food sources.

In the Upper-Right quadrant, they suggest that we eat optimal foods. In other words, the authors suggest that we do our research and find out what diets work the best for us. For example, some people actually need red meat, while others don't. Some people seem to be able to get by on a vegetarian diet, while this doesn't seem to work for others. There are many contradictory schools and theories of nutrition. I recommend that you consciously and mindfully explore this field to find the diet that works best for you. Take your time, be aware, and experiment. For example, if a heavy lunch of pasta puts you to sleep for three hours, you might want to try something else. Be aware, too, that as we change and age, or increase or decrease our physical activity, our dietary needs will change over time.

As I said at the beginning of the chapter, nutrition is foundational. When you learn to "eat to live" rather than live to eat, you will quickly see improvement in the amount of energy you have, in your well-being, in the lifting of general feelings of depression and sluggishness, in your strength during your workouts, and in the clarity of your mind in your meditation. Remember, your body is the temple of your spirit and the vehicle of your life.

To end this discussion, I would like to recommend the following books by some of the pioneers in the field of nutritional recovery:

Beasley, Joseph D., M.D. *Food for Recovery.* New York: Crown, 1994.

Cousens, Gabriel, M.D. *Depression-Free for Life.* New York: HarperCollins, 2000.

D'Adamo, Peter J., Dr. *Eat Right 4 Your Type.* New York: Putnam's Sons, 1996.

Larson, Joan Mathews, Ph.D. *Seven Weeks to Sobriety.* New York: Ballantine, 1997.

Larson, Joan Mathews, Ph.D. *Depression-Free, Naturally.* New York: Ballantine, 1999.

Lesser, Michael, M.D. *The Brain Chemistry Diet.* New York: Putnam's Sons, 2002.

Newport, John, Ph.D. *The Wellness-Recovery Connection*. Deerfield Beach: Health Communications, Inc., 2004.

Sears, Barry, Ph.D. *Enter the Zone*. New York: HarperCollins, 1995.

Sears, Barry, Ph.D. *Mastering the Zone*. New York: HarperCollins, 1997.

Slaga, Thomas J., and Robin Keuneke. *The Detox Revolution*. New York: McGraw-Hill Books, 2003.

Weil, Andrew, M.D. *Eating Well for Optimum Health*. New York: Knopf, 2000.

9

Transforming the Brain

It was early on in my quest for an Integral Recovery model that I first heard about binaural brainwave entrainment technology. While listening to some collected conversations on the Integral website, Integralnaked. org, I came across three conversations with Bill Harris and Ken Wilber, in which they discussed brainwave entrainment in general, and specifically the technology Harris had developed at Centerpointe Research Institute, called Holosync®. I was intrigued. Harris claimed that his technology allows us to replicate or even exceed the brainwave states of the most experienced and dedicated meditators. Not only that, but in short order the user of this technology starts to experience the myriad positive effects of a profound prolonged meditation practice, not in years, but in days or weeks. These effects include the following:

- reduced stress, including reduced production of the negative brain chemicals cortisol and CRF, which figure so largely in producing cravings in the addict's brain;

- deep relaxation;

- increased IQ;

- enhanced creativity;

- accelerated spiritual growth;

- accelerated learning;

- increased memory;

- occurrence of peak performance states;

- elimination of substance abuse problems;

- alleviation of depression and anxiety;

- change and elimination of unwanted habits and attitudes;

- release of trauma, coupled with reowning split-off shadow elements in the psyche;

- rapid development of the Transcendent Witness/observer self.

The instructions were simple: just listen to a CD with stereo headphones for an hour every day, paying attention to whatever is happening while you listen. On the first track, you hear the sound of rain and what sounds like glass bowls ringing. On the second track, you hear just the rain. All you hear are the pleasant sounds. The real work is happening subsonically underneath the rain and ringing. In the left ear, there is one beat, in the right ear, another. Most people can't hear them, but the brain does. The brain can't handle the discrepancy in the two different beats, say 100 and 110 beats per minute, so it splits the difference to a "phantom" beat of, say, 5 hertz. This entrains your brain waves at the very low brainwave state of 5 hertz. In this case of 5 hertz, the corresponding brainwave state is theta, the state associated with REM/dream sleep.

This promised to be too good to be true. Being a skeptic, I began researching and gathering data from the internet. I found out that brainwave entrainment was not a new technology; it had been around since at least 1973, and perhaps much longer.

The History of Binaural Brainwave Entrainment Meditation

During the 1970s, Western scientists began investigating the effects of meditation and using as their subjects experienced long-term meditators such as swamis, nuns, and monks—people with years of experience in a monastic practice, who meditated daily. What they found, to their surprise, was that these experienced meditators could actually change their brainwave states through the conscious effort of meditation. This was a revelation to the scientists, as not only had they suspected that meditation was merely a premodern, superstitious practice, but it was also commonly believed that brain waves were not controllable; they were perceived as acting somewhat like the weather, coming and going and doing whatever they wanted. Discovering that brainwave states could be consciously manipulated led to a renaissance in meditation research and a deeper understanding of the brain and our potential for transformative meditation and growth.

In 1973, Dr. Gerald Oster, of the Mt. Sinai Medical Center, published a paper in the October issue of *Scientific American*. In this paper, entitled *Auditory Beats in the Brain,* Dr. Oster explained how, by putting differing beats in each ear using stereo headphones, he was able to entrain the brain to whatever brainwave state was desired. For example, if he played 100 beats (or hertz) into the left ear and 110 into the right ear, the brain, not knowing how to deal with this discrepancy, would split the difference, creating a phantom beat not at 105 hertz but at 5 hertz, which, in this case, plants you in a theta brainwave state. Now previously it had been thought that only through disciplined monastic daily meditative practice, for five, ten, or fifteen years, could you consciously change your brainwave state into a deep meditative state. Dr. Oster found that anyone can change his brainwave state—even the man off the street—almost immediately using binaural beats. Not only can you change your brain waves to a desired state, but you can also remain in that state for as long as you want. This was the beginning of the binaural revolution.

What early researchers had found with the most advanced of meditators was that they could spike their brainwave states into the deep meditative states of theta and delta, usually just for brief periods. Using binaural meditation, however, it was quite easy to keep the brain waves of binaural meditators stable in these deep states for as long as was desired. What happens when this is achieved is revolutionary and transformational: what appears to happen when the brain is kept in these deep states for extended periods in a daily practice is that the brain is pushed beyond its current functioning capacity and actually transforms. In a strictly material, neurological sense, this looks like increased neuronal growth, brain cell growth, more optimal neurochemical balance (such as increased dopamine and serotonin levels and decreased cortisol), the development of new neural pathways, and the balancing of the functions of the left and right hemispheres of the brain.

What this means, for the purposes of Integral Recovery, is that we can now induce deep transformative brainwave states almost immediately in recovering addicts from day one. Not only can we induce these states, but what occurs is that recovering addicts begin to experience the fruits of deep meditative practice in a very short period of time. These benefits include feelings of serenity, mental clarity, and relief of stress, among other

Awakening Both of Your Brains

We are living in the "Golden Age" of brain research, and what has become apparent is that we really have two brains, a right and a left, more commonly called the right and left hemispheres. The left brain generally deals with linear, analytical issues, and the right brain deals with more intuitive ways of knowing. If we take pictures of someone's brain at any given time, using an EEG, for example, we would find that people are generally right-brain or left-brain dominant. Left-brain-dominant people tend to be more focused on exteriors—out there in the world and getting things done—while right-brain-dominant people are more focused on interiors—intuitive, or spiritual, if you will. The left brain functions in a more classically masculine way of perception and the right brain in a more feminine manner. This is rather astounding; a masculine/feminine or assertive/receptive brain.

What makes this so fascinating for our work is that studies have shown that after using Holosync® for a while, both sides of the brain come online equally.[1] A metaphor I use to explain what this feels like is to imagine that you have only been looking at the world through one eye. Go ahead, cover one of your eyes and look around. You will notice that everything appears flat with no depth. Now remove your hand from the covered eye and look out of both of them. You will notice that there is a great change, everything is in 3D, and everything has new depth. This is what it is like when your two brain hemispheres begin to sync up and work together. There is a new depth to your life. You are no longer a square but a cube.

things. By accessing and staying in theta, deep theta, and particularly delta states, we can release our deepest traumas, access our highest self, tap into our creativity, and connect experientially with our deepest spiritual self. In addition to this, most people find the experience of binaurally enhanced meditation quite pleasurable, which means that with a little coaching and inspiration, people tend to stick with the practice. This in itself is huge. Before using binaural methods, I spent years attempting to get my beloved addicts to meditate, with very little success.

Another aspect of our healing work at these deep states of consciousness is that visualizations and affirmations become very powerful and effective. A case in point is the ground-breaking work of Dr. Eugene Peniston and Dr. Paul Kulkowski at the University of Southern Colorado in 1989.[2] They selected a group of forty late-stage alcoholics who had been in jail or prison more than once due to their drinking. Twenty of this group went through standard treatment: 12-step work, meetings, and individual counseling. The other twenty were given fifteen neurofeedback sessions in which they were trained to slow their brains down to deep theta. Then they were given visualizations and affirmations.

The progress of these two groups was tracked over a ten-year period. At the end of ten years, eighteen out of the twenty alcoholics who went through standard treatment had relapsed, and most were dead. Out of the twenty who had done the neurofeedback work, the affirmations and the visualizations, eighteen were still sober and tested very positively in a battery of psychological tests measuring happiness, purpose, quality of relationships, and so on. "This group showed a marked personality transformation, including significant increases in qualities such as warmth, stability, conscientiousness, boldness, imaginativeness, and self-control, along with decreases in depression and anxiety."[3] Imagine what kind of results we can get if our Integral Recovery practitioners have access to these same states, not fifteen times, but for an hour every day for the rest of their lives!

In general, binaural brainwave entrainment technologies have been specifically designed to take the listener from beta, the normal walk-around consciousness, down into deep delta. This is interesting, because most research done with expert meditators shows that these meditators spike briefly into theta waves. What we have found with binaural brainwave entrainment is that the even deeper brainwave state delta is more powerful and transformative than theta, delta being a frequency that most of the time even the most experienced meditators cannot reach through their own traditional meditative practices. In the beginning years of binaural brainwave entrainment use and experimentation, it was initially thought that alpha was the optimal state to which to entrain the brain. Then, over time, theta became the brain wave of choice for a transformational, meditative, auditory track. However, eventually it was understood that the lowest brainwave frequency, or delta, was the most efficacious or powerful for achieving the aforementioned desired results.

With this technology, we are not only able to reach delta brainwave states, but also to stay in them for extended periods of time.

As I described in chapter 5 ("Integrating Healthy States of Consciousness"), if you can imagine brain waves as wavy lines, beta is the fastest frequency with the smallest, shallowest waves. As you progress into alpha, then theta, and finally delta, there are fewer waves, but they are more powerful. The slower and larger the waves, the more powerful they are and the more they push the brain to grow and reorganize at a higher level of integration and functioning.

In my own life (and I have heard similar stories from many of my students and Profound Meditation Program users), my capacity to gracefully handle situations that used to overwhelm me has grown remarkably. For many years, I suffered from ongoing cycles and bouts of crippling depression, where an event or a series of events would happen that would throw me into a seriously depressed state that would sometimes last for months. During this time, I was often incapacitated in my ability to work and hold down a job and was frequently experiencing suicidal thoughts, where death seemed a welcome release from the depths of my suffering. Since I began my Integral practice, of which binaurally enhanced meditation is a central part, that which used to knock me off my center and throw me into the deep pits of my depression and despair no longer does.

Far from being guarded or immune from deeply feeling the events in my life, I now feel them more deeply and more fully; I open to and accept feelings that arise, with an understanding that they are not to be avoided, run from, or medicated, but simply allowed to express themselves. Sometimes, I have experienced a day or two of feeling deep and painful emotions, but now I have the capacity to let them be, and they pass much more quickly. So instead of being terrified of these deep and often distressing feelings, for fear that I would be thrown into another major episode of clinical depression, I have learned that they come and they go and that there are actually extremely beneficial effects of allowing these feelings to be experienced and accepted.

For example, if sadness is the issue that emerges during your meditation or in the rest of your life, the way to work with the sadness is to embrace it and absolutely accept it. Any attempt to avoid the sadness or to try to make yourself "happy" is contraindicated and harmful. The sadness is there for a reason, and it must be allowed to express itself sensationally in your body. This does not mean that your cognitive interpretations about the causes of the sadness are necessarily correct or in some sense ultimately true, but the feelings are real and must be honored and express themselves, so the energy can be released, and you can move on. For example, you might be feeling sad because you think that everyone thinks you're an idiot, when the truth might be that everyone thinks you are brilliant. In this case, the sadness is real, but your understanding is off; still, the bodily feelings must be honored and validated. It is when we try to avoid our emotions and our negative feelings that we begin to get stuck and create new pathologies or add to our old ones. So when you are sad, allow yourself to be sad. Deeply feel the feelings, and they will come, and they will pass.

Let's look at something that may seem paradoxical. On the one hand, stress is public enemy number one, on the other hand, it is stress that pushes us to grow and evolve. Using the definition of stress provided by pioneering scientist Dr. Selye,[4] we can differentiate between two types of stress: distress and eustress. Distress is negative stress, which will weaken our immune system, age us prematurely, and begin the compulsive cravings that lead to relapse. But we also have eustress, or positive stress, which will cause a system to transform and grow. A physical example of this would be when we work out with progressively heavier weights during our strength training, the muscles are stressed temporarily and break down, only to grow back stronger.

The same thing happens in our binaurally enhanced meditation work: as the carrier frequencies become progressively lower (the neurological equivalent of adding more weight in the gym), we are pushed to ever higher levels of neurological functioning and growth. In the Upper-Right quadrant, this looks like a healthier, more optimally functioning brain; in the Upper-Left quadrant, the interior, this feels like more capacity to deal with life and suffering, more creativity, more serenity, higher cognitive functioning, and definitely more sobriety. Over time, many people report a gradual sense of increasing access to an intuitive sense of inner wisdom and guidance. (See the highly recommended book *Living Deeply*, based on a 10-year study by the Institute of Noetic Sciences on what constitutes transformation and the fruits of transformation.)

Binaurally enhanced meditation puts us through progressive experiences of chaos, thereby initiating reorganization at a higher level. If we freak out when this begins to happen, take off the headphones, and head for the hills, reorganization at a higher level will not happen. Therefore, we must embrace this experience of chaos, or positive stress, in the moment. What happens after this reorganization is allowed to occur is that at the new higher level of organization, the things that used to anger us and cause us stress simply don't bother us as much anymore. This is what is called raising the stress threshold.

My Journey with Binaural Brainwave Entrainment

I want to briefly relate my own initial experience with binaurally enhanced meditation, in order to give you a general idea of what can happen. Very quickly in the first week, I began to experience a profound and peaceful spaciousness in my meditation. Thoughts and emotions would arise, but they arose as objects in a vast ocean of peace, or, for lack of a better word, bliss. I soon noticed that this "Witness" became available also when I was not meditating. For example, I could be having an argument with my wife, and a part of me would observe myself arguing. My experience was, "Wow, part of me is absolutely free; I can choose to continue this argument with gusto or just laugh, hug my wife, or whatever, but I am free!" Good old John is still hanging in there doing his thing, but the deeper me is vast and free and watching the whole show. It's the difference between playing Macbeth and forgetting you're acting, and thinking that you are Macbeth. Thinking you *are* Macbeth can be a pretty tragic affair; however, playing Macbeth can be a heck of a lot of fun.

A Chopped Finger and Scary Monsters

I had two very powerful dreams in this initial phase, which bear telling. But before I get started, let me say that probably 80 percent of the people I have worked with, who use this type of enhanced meditation, reported powerful dreams and a much more vivid dream life altogether. In the first couple of weeks of my binaural practice, I had the following two dreams.

The first one took place in the building that housed Passages to Recovery (one of the therapeutic wilderness programs I helped found). A group of us was inside the building, but it was stripped and in the process of being renovated. I was working with a saw, and I suddenly cut off the tip of my little finger, a very small piece. In the dream, this really upset me. I went to my wife, Pam, who was busy working on something else, and said, "Honey, I cut off the tip of my finger!" She responded, "That's nice," and kept working. Nobody seemed to care. I was really upset.

In the next scene, I was at the local clinic, holding the tip of my finger. I went to the woman at the desk and said, "I cut off the tip of my finger!" She responded with something like, "That's nice, sir. Take a seat." At this point, I was ready to cry. Nobody cared! Then I dropped the tip of my finger on the floor and looked at it. I shrugged and thought, "It's just the tip of my little finger." At that moment, I shot through the roof of the clinic, like a shell fired out of a cannon vertically, flying with great force and speed up into the clouds, where there were great flashes of lightning and explosions of thunder! I woke up with my heart pounding, shocked by the intensity of the experience.

The meaning of the dream soon became clear: The tip of my little finger was my ego self—just the smallest fraction of who and what I really am. As soon as I stopped worrying about it so much and put it in a more realistic perspective, the vertical growth I experienced was astronomical.

The second dream, following shortly on the heels of the first, went as follows. I was in Houston, Texas, in one of the houses I grew up in. The house was full of family members. I looked out of the back window and saw huge, prehistoric, armadillo-like monsters walking down the street. They were BIG—twice as tall as the house, and longer than a semitruck hauling a trailer. My first reaction was terror, and I felt an urge to move my family to the center of the house. Then I was observing the enormous creatures from the window of my bedroom, as they passed in the front of my house. The next thing I knew, I was running toward these monsters and then vaulting over them like one of the dancers or athletes pictured in ancient Cretan artwork, who vault over ferocious-looking bulls. Strangely enough, I was starting to have fun. And each time I vaulted over one of the creatures, it began to shrink. By the time the dream ended, they were as small as Volkswagons, and I was having a grand time playing with them. Again, the meaning of the dream soon became clear. The big, scary monsters were my own rejected shadows and wounds, which I had been running from for years. But as soon as I began to deal with them creatively and playfully, their menace greatly diminished, and my experience actually became joyful and fun.

Why am I recounting these dreams? Because the wisdom they contain became a guide to my own personal growth and healing processes. The same thing frequently happens with my clients, for whom potent and instructive dreams tend to emerge within the first few days of beginning this practice. Over the last six years, my dream life has remained very powerful and often lucid. In other words, I am often aware I am dreaming while I am dreaming. This seems to be a common occurrence among those who are using this technology.

I encourage those of you who are doing this work to pay attention to your dreams. It is helpful to have a journal next to your bed, in which you can make notes about your dreams, or even a recording device, so you can record your dreams as soon as possible upon awakening, because in most cases the memories will fade if not recorded promptly. A big mistake we can make with our dreams is to say, oh, that was stupid, and dismiss them. In our dreams we have access to our deep selves, and often our issues, which can largely be unconscious, are revealed through the symbolic images of our dreams. Dreams will disclose answers to our unresolved issues, directions for our soul's journey, and contain the seeds of our creativity. There also seems to be an energy, a vitality, contained in dreams that gets released as we work with them and begin to understand them.

I was recently reading an autobiography of Keith Richards, the Rolling Stones guitarist and songwriter. He related how he kept a tape recorder next to his bed to record his dreams. One morning, he noticed that the tape recorder had been used overnight. He rewound the tape and listened, and, behold, there was the song, (I can't get no) "Satisfaction." The rest, as they say, is history. This song became a smash hit for the Rolling Stones, and to this day it is a rock and roll classic.

I often work with my dreams as I am doing my morning BWE meditation. I will simply review the dream and feel the emotions that the images and story evoke and stay with that, often with quite amazing results. The point here is that this type of meditation will enhance your dream life and give you new tools for healing and creativity.

Back to my story. As I continued to practice binaural meditation, following this initial, powerful, spiritual opening, I began a nine-month period of intense emotional release and healing. During my daily meditation practice, I experienced strong emotional upheavals, often accompanied by mounting pain or discomfort in my heart area or gut. In the new context of my developing ability to shift into a Witness or observer, I allowed the pain to be there without resisting it or pushing it away. I allowed the bodily sensations to grow, or stay, or change, or whatever would happen, while I just watched them with alertness and curiosity.

I also noted cognitive messages that came with these feelings. If I was dealing with traumatic, repressed material, the message would be along the order of, "This is too much! If you go into this darkness, it will destroy you! Do something else . . . This is too frightening." But I was able to simply bracket such thoughts and think, "These are only thoughts, stories, interpretations—my self-created fictions." I let them arise, then be, and then pass on. I did not let them run the show, but I allowed them to be there as part of the gestalt of the traumatic material that was emerging. Often, as the bodily felt sensations emerged and strengthened, the thoughts and associated stories got more desperate: "No, no, you really can't go here!" I realized that these were the very voices and thoughts inhibiting my further growth, healing, and happiness, the ones that would keep me stuck.

Often, I watched all of the mental, emotional, and bodily felt sensations build into a crescendo and then they would release. After the release, I felt an inner spaciousness, serenity, and even a blissful joy. Frequently, this release would be followed by a deep intuitive understanding of what had transpired, compassion for myself and others, forgiveness for others, forgiveness of myself, and with all of that, a tremendous energy and aliveness was released into my life. My inner battle cry became, "They are just feelings!" As I plunged ever more deeply into my being, I learned that all of these traumas, dragons, and monsters were merely surfaces that I could confront, dialogue with, and release. This was a tremendous realization and breakthrough in my personal journey and is now one of the essential components of Integral Recovery.

The above is part of my story, but, over the years, I have collected and heard so many stories of revelation and transformation from those who are using binaural brainwave entrainment technology as an ongoing daily practice, that at some point they could be a book in themselves. For now, I will relate just one of those stories, which is interesting because of the individual's youth and lack of prior knowledge of the technology and its effects.

This is what happened with a young friend of mine. I'll call him Tom. Tom is seventeen years old, a junior in high school, an athlete, and someone with whom I occasionally work out at my local gym. I gave Tom a binaural CD track and told him to try listening to it for a few days, after which I left town on a trip. About three weeks later, I saw Tom at the gym and asked him if had tried the CD. A look of wonder crossed his face, and he told me his story. I asked him to write his experience down, and this is what he wrote: "I've been pretty amazed at how this has been working. I listen to this every morning before school for a half hour; it has worked wonders. I have experienced viewing things at different angles, and getting a better understanding of everything. My grades in school have gone up exceedingly, and I am a lot more focused and patient."

I had told Tom very little about what to expect. He just did the practice. Tom is experiencing his world with more depth and with a brain that, in a very short time, had begun to function at a higher level. In my work with adolescents, I have noticed that young people seem to be especially sensitive to this technology and experience the positive benefits very quickly.

It is my hope that you who are reading this chapter will be inspired to adopt brainwave entrainment as an ongoing healing and transformative practice in your lives. I have often thought that if this book had no other effect than to promote the use of brainwave entrainment technology as an accepted part of addiction treatment, that in itself would be more than enough.[5]

An interesting unfoldment of this history happened after I had completed the final draft of the *Integral Recovery* manuscript. I was on a business trip to Boulder, Colorado, and a friend who knew of my interest in and use of binaural technology introduced me to Eric Thompson. Eric told me how much this technology had changed his life and helped him with his depression and I shared my story. Eric said that at a certain point, he had felt a calling to work to improve this technology and that he had created a more effective and powerful technology than the one we had both been using. Eric did this by improving the binaural entrainment process itself and by layering other transformational technologies into the audio tracks he was producing. This sounded good to me but I was, quite frankly, a bit skeptical.

Eric then provided me with some of the tracks he was creating and I told him I would try them out. I had been using brainwave entrainment technology on a daily basis for around five years at this point and had developed a high sensitivity to my own inner states and a connoisseur's appreciation of the different brainwave entrainment technologies that were available at the time. Upon listening to Eric's tracks, I immediately felt their power and efficacy and got back with Eric. We decided to throw in our lots together, and, along with my wife Pam, developed the company iAwake Technologies, whose leading product is the Profound

Meditation Program. As of this writing, iAwake Technologies has been going for two years and the community of users is expanding around the globe. The results that we personally have been experiencing, and what we have heard from those who are using the Profound Meditation Program, have been nothing short of amazing.

Recharging the Brain with Cranial Electrical Stimulation

Another very exciting technology that Integral Recovery includes is cranial electrical stimulation (CES). This technology has been around a long time, since the first decade of the twentieth century. There have been at least 110 clinical studies on CES conducted in the United States and many more in Europe and Russia.[6] The results of these studies are amazing. Among the notable conditions that are greatly improved are chronic pain, anxiety, depression, insomnia, headaches, and muscle tension, as well as cravings for drugs and withdrawal symptoms.

Generally, this technology has been utilized with earlobe clips; however, more recently, I have begun to use a new and improved version called the Fisher Wallace Stimulator. Instead of earlobe clips, the Fisher Wallace Stimulator uses an elastic headband with two plates fronted by sponges, which administer gentle electrical charges transcranially, or, in other words, directly through the skull into the brain. I am now recommending this device for all my students, as it seems to be more effective and even more powerful than the earlier versions I used. The practice is to put on the headband, wet the sponges to aid the conductivity, and turn on the handheld device powered by two AA batteries. Upon turning on the Stimulator, one feels a slight tingle in the temples, and after twenty minutes, the device turns off automatically. I currently have my students use the Stimulator twice a day, during both their morning and afternoon meditation sessions. This practice is carried out for the first 45 days of treatment. After that, I recommend my students use the device a few times a month, and perhaps after three months, repeat the 45-day process.[7]

So what, actually, is this technology doing? There are numerous schools of thought on this, so I will describe the two major ones. The first says that CES stimulates the hypothalamus of the brain, which is the area in charge of releasing hormones and regulating neurochemicals, such as serotonin, dopamine, norepinephrine, CRF, and cortisol. CES decreases cortisol and CRF, which are stress-related neurochemicals associated with depression, anxiety, and increased cravings for drugs, and greatly increases the bioavailability of the other beneficial neurochemicals in the brain. Not only that, but this all apparently happens almost immediately.

One of the problems with antidepressants of the selective serotonin reuptake inhibitors (SSRI) variety specifically, is that they take weeks and sometimes months to work—if they do. This simply is not good enough if one is severely depressed or going through withdrawal from drugs. With CES, the relief is felt quite quickly. If one is, for example, using CES while withdrawing from heroin, the withdrawal symptoms, the bad feelings, and the anxieties are significantly decreased. It is truly extraordinary. Other benefits of CES technology are increased cognitive function, greater concentration (good for ADHD sufferers), enhanced memory, and positive personality transformation.

The second school of thought is that CES simply charges and energizes the whole brain to function at a much higher level.

I would definitely recommend CES as the option of first choice before taking antidepressants. There are no negative side effects from using CES, and, unlike antidepressants, it seems to be "unabusable," in that once optimal neurobiological balance has been established, it won't continue to produce more and more neurochemicals. It simply stops doing anything. A metaanalysis of antidepressant drugs and CES out of Europe showed CES to be 70 percent more effective than the most effective antidepressant drug, Paxil.[8] If you are interested in reading more of the clinical information, I recommend the Fisher Wallace and the Alpha-Stim websites, which contain a number of good clinical studies on the efficacy of CES for various afflictions.[9] In terms of sheer cost effectiveness, the cost of one of these devices is far lower than the cost of being on antidepressant drugs for a year.

In Integral Recovery Practice, we use CES along with our meditation for the first 20 minutes of our 40-minute morning meditation and for all of the 20-minute evening meditation. Many of my students have noted that meditations using binaural technology and CES simultaneously tend to become even deeper than normal.

I have found that BWE technology and CES technology do many of the same things: they produce healthy neurochemical balance, alleviate depression and anxiety, and cause the brain to function at a higher level. I have not found that CES allows for the emotional release work and the spiritual depth work that BWE technology does, but used together, as with all of our IR practices, they seem to synergize each other, both working more effectively. Another real plus is that one can use this at home, without going to a hospital surrounded by professionals in white lab coats. This allows for a very positive sense of ownership and control of one's own recovery process. It might seem a little silly at first, with the headphones and ear clips, or elastic headbands with sponges and wires, but, what the heck, it is a small price to pay, and it works.

On a last note, you might ask, "Well, if this is so effectual, and so cost effective, why isn't it being used more?" To spare the reader from a paranoid-sounding rant, I will simply say that most likely there are financial interests at stake here. CES is approved by the FDA as a treatment for depression, anxiety, and pain, and the United States is the only country in the world that requires CES to be prescribed by a healthcare professional. This can be a physician's assistant, a nurse, a doctor, or a rehab specialist. One should not have any problem finding an enlightened U.S. healthcare professional to prescribe CES. These devices can also be ordered off the internet without a prescription, if you are outside of the United States.

As stated earlier in this book, one of the truly terrible things about addiction is that addicts soon become anhedonic through their use of drugs or alcohol. This means that in the absence of the drug, they are unable to experience pleasure. With CES, anhedonia is quickly alleviated, and the addict is able, once again, to feel good and experience pleasure in the normal things of life without using drugs. This is a breakthrough of great promise in the treatment of addiction and should go a long way toward easing the suffering associated with recovery, leading to increased sobriety, with far fewer incidences of relapse. It is extremely helpful in early recovery, as the recovering addict begins to feel good and to feel relief almost immediately. This, of course, allows for more effective progress in all the essential lines and quadrants. The feeling that "I'm getting better" and even *life* is getting better is a major turning point in treatment.

CES is not a silver bullet and will not by itself cure addiction. However, it is a powerful tool that should become one of the basic treatments used in the recovery field and certainly deserves to be one of our top treatment modalities in the Integral Recovery model.

Epigenetics: Inspiration from the Cutting Edge of Science

And now for something really exciting and paradigm shattering. The Human Genome Project was initiated in 1990 and largely completed by 2003. The findings are fascinating as, in the beginning, it was estimated that the human genome would consist of perhaps two million genes, but what geneticists discovered was that it consists of merely 20,000 to 25,000 genes. Many had thought that the mapping of the human genome was the holy grail of scientific understanding of the building blocks of life and that once that was completed, we would have figured out the basis of biological human life itself and could all go home and take a nap. Well, it turns out that this was just the beginning of our understanding. As recently as the year 2000, the term "epigenetics" was coined—epi meaning "above"—and what this new science of epigenetics has begun to explore is how our 25,000 or so genes express themselves.[10]

The fact that the number of genes was so low, around 25,000, puzzled scientists, because this did not seem like enough to account for something as complex as the human brain. (Amazingly, scientists have found that fruit flies and ringworm have nearly as large a genome as humans; the human genome is less than a factor of two greater than the genome of fruit flies and ringworm.) What scientists then began to discover was that the genes themselves were something like a hard drive that stored information and that what was ultimately responsible for our physical and emotional conditioning was not so much the genes themselves but how they express themselves moment to moment. Imagine having an alphabet with 25,000 letters and the different combinations of letters and meaning that could be produced from such a large alphabet. Hello, genome!

What scientists are now finding in this new field of scientific inquiry is shattering our old genetic paradigm, which went something like this: You are dealt a hand of genetic cards from your parents, and you gotta play the hand you are dealt. If you have addict genes, you are likely to become an addict. Deal with it. If you have depressed genes, you'll be depressed. If you have dumb genes, you'll be dumb, and so on. Not very exciting unless you have really smart and beautiful parents. Very deterministic. Not very hopeful. What science is now saying is that our genetic inheritance is responsible for only about 10 percent of our condition. The other 90 percent is absolutely responsive to our environment, and not just over long periods of time but from moment to moment![11]

By environment, scientists mean both our inner and our outer environments, or, in Integral speak, all four quadrants. So, this means the expression of our genes = genes x environment. In other words, our environment, which controls the expression of our genes—whether we are healthy, happy, smart, or sober—is under *our* control in the form of the thoughts we think, the foods we eat, the practices we do, the relationships we have, the homes we live in, the organizations we belong to, and so on. What this science also shows us is that if, for example, you have addict genes from, say, your grandfather, and indeed are an addict, but then you go into recovery, you will pass on that recovery capacity epigenetically to your children.

I'll give an example, a true story, of how this might play out. (This is strictly my interpretation of the new scientific story that is emerging.) I have a friend, whose early career consisted of being an out-of-control, alcoholic drug addict, given to rage and violence, who, in fact, spent time in a state penitentiary. During this period, he was married and had a family. The children of his marriage reflect the epigenetic expression of my friend's genes at that time and have all been severely troubled. However, he did eventually clean up his act and launched a remarkable career helping others. He also had a second marriage and a second family. The children of his second marriage were remarkably healthy and well adapted.

While there are obviously multiple factors affecting the children of both of these marriages, it is very easy to extrapolate that the genetic expression my friend donated to his second family was a much healthier version than his earlier genetic expression. What this says to us, individually and collectively, is, "Get busy! Take responsibility. Create health and hope in how you live your lives and practice from moment to moment, day to day, month to month, and year to year!" We are creating our biological future, not as guinea pigs or victims, but as the owners and guardians of our own genes and their expression.

The clear moral inference in this case is *responsibility*. We are responsible for our own genes and how they express themselves in our lives. This adds even more weight to our insistence, in Integral Recovery, that all four quadrants are included in the recovery process and that Integral Recovery Practice becomes central to our lives, because our thoughts and attitudes control our genetic expression. Our dietary choices control our genetic expression; our meditations, mindfulness, and shadow practices control our genetic expression; our skillfulness in handling the various emotional states that arise from moment to moment controls our genetic expression; our relationships with others and our environment, affected by the alchemical mystery of mirror neurons,[12] control our genetic expression; our exercise controls our genetic expression; and, perhaps even more important, our *intentionality* controls our genetic expression.

We are moving from a world where we are acted upon by the environment, passive victims of our genes, to a world that we are co-creating through our intentionality, conscious practices, and conscious ability to heal and transform the world inside and outside of us. We are no longer merely the products of some impersonal, random process of evolution and natural selection, but are moving into a new epoch of co-creating and conscious evolution that transpires from moment to moment to moment. In other words, if you don't like your genes, fix them. About 90 percent of that is on your shoulders. No more whining; no more excuses; get with it, get well, stay with it, and evolve now.

Taking responsibility for our genetic expression also determines the genetic inheritance of the generations that come after us. Because what appears to be emerging in our understanding of the dynamics of epigenetics is that we pass on not only the hard-drive genetic structure but also the genetic expressions. So our healthy attitudes, our practices, our healthy diets, and all that we have struggled to establish in our lives actually become easier for, and passed on to, those who come after us. Much as the sins of the father, to quote the Bible, are passed on from generation to generation, our healthy habits, intentions, and attitudes are also transferred from generation to generation.

In order to illustrate this point and the importance of practice, which can be defined as cultivation through repetition, I will quote from the writings of Dawson Church's book *The Genie in Your Genes: Epigenetic Medicine and the New Biology of Intention*.[13] Eric Kandel, M.D., who received the Nobel Prize of Medicine in 2000, says that learning produces change in people by "producing changes in gene expression that alter the strength of synaptic connections, and structural changes that alter the anatomical patterns of interconnections between nerve cells of the brain." In one experiment, Kandel discovered that when new memories are established, the number of synaptic connections in the sensory neurons that were stimulated jumped to around 2,600, a doubling of its previous count of 1,300. Unless the initial experience was reinforced, however, the number of connections dropped back to 1,300 within three weeks. If we reinforce our novel experiences by repetition, we strengthen the neural net to support them; if we do not, our newfound neural circuitry quickly decays—not over years, but in less than a month. This means that new thoughts, actions, and habits (practices!) must be continuously updated in order to take root.

This sheds new light on our recognition that simply going to treatment for 28 days or 3 months is not enough. What continues and reinforces the new synaptic pathways, new attitudes, new intentions, and new health is the cultivation through repetition, or practice, of the essential Integral Recovery practices that keep us healthy, transforming, and evolving over the now potentially ever-increasing span of our lives. George Leonard, in his classic work *Mastery*, tells us what kind of practices do not work: the Hacker, the Dabbler, and the Obsessive do not reach mastery. The Obsessive wants the transformation now and does not stick with it. The Dabbler merely dabbles, as in "I went to the gym twice and it didn't do anything." And the Hacker is satisfied with plateaus and does not keep pushing his practice to new levels of depth and excellence. The Master, however, stays with the practice for a lifetime, through peak experiences, through new plateaus, and into the area of lasting, long-term transformation and optimal genetic expression.[14] Recall again that Integral Recovery Practice is not just a call to exercise one skill or one practice, but a practice that covers all of the essential territories so that our transformation is holistic, balanced, and almost infinitely nuanced and dynamic.

Much of my work, as it has emerged in the last few years with new students, is simply being an auxiliary superego[15] for the first few weeks, in order to harangue, cajole, inspire, and hold students accountable to do their daily practices. After a few weeks or a month, the seed begins to germinate and take root, and the recovery process takes on a new energy coming from the individual herself. When the dynamic of the process of transformation, brought about by Integral practice, starts becoming clear to the student, the motivation and discipline become self-generated and, behold, we have a new master, one who sticks with the practice. As practice continues, and our understanding of our responsibility to heal, transform, self-actualize, and ultimately Self-realize deepens, the journey truly becomes the destination itself. Radical evolutionary crescendos are accepted with the same equanimity as the more subtle plateau periods. On and on, our practice deepens with an ever-increasing ability to appreciate the subtleties as well as the vastly apparent shifts—the big "Aha!" moments.

To illustrate how this consistency to practice showed its fruits in my life, I will give you an example. As a buildup, perhaps, to this period of writing, I went through two weeks of profound pain and suffering in my practice, especially in my meditational practice. What I noticed, after a while, though, was my ability to be present with the darkness and with the suffering. A small part of me wanted to run for the hills from the darkness, but the larger, more dominant part of me, which I call my "surrender muscles," could and would do nothing but surrender to the process. This surrender began to take on an almost effortless quality. Coming from a place a few years ago of "I don't surrender to anybody, anyway, anyhow," this shows a remarkable transformation brought on by years of practice and the struggle to hold my deepest and most profound suffering in awareness. What are the results of this capacity to surrender to suffering in my practice? A deeper sense of connection to myself, my loved ones, my students, my world, and also deep humility, mixed with a sense of hope and gratitude, for the grace and the mystery of my life.

These sorts of results take patience, time, and persistence. Although this transformational process is rapid indeed, and often dramatically so, it does take time and stick-to-it-ness. In the early stages of recovery, some of my students are impatient, easily frustrated, and want immediate results. As their practice deepens, however, they become able to watch the quick-fix, demanding addict part of themselves, the one who wants immediate gratification, and that, too, becomes grist for the mill, as mindfulness and compassion begin to transform the incessant demands, anger, and cravings of the addicted self. To paraphrase one of the principal slogans of IR, "Relapse happens when we stop practicing," we could say, "Relapse happens when we do not reinforce our newly emergent synaptic pathways and positively reinforce our genetic expression from moment to moment, hour to hour, and day to day."

10

Healing the Emotions and the
Power of the Shadow

While all of the core Integral Recovery Practices dealing with body, mind, spirit, and shadow work together in a cross-training, synergistic fashion, there's a particular alliance between spirit and emotion/shadow work. That's because the spiritual experience of meditation often brings the practitioner face to face with a slew of inner demons that need to be dealt with. Since addictive behavior in large part consists of running away from self-awareness and emotional integrity, this emotion/shadow work is an especially important front in the battle for recovery. As we learn to hold our issues and our egos in an ever-larger context, they don't go "poof!" and disappear in a single blaze of glory, but they do become lighter and lighter. We become less fearful and attached as we move through and release our old knots, traumas, and conditioning. The alternative is to stay stuck in our old conditioned patterns of understanding and behavior, which is exactly what we want to avoid. Eventually our emotional triggers lose their hold over us, and with that goes their power to cause relapse and suffering.

Pure witnessing (or seeing and identifying one's issues through meditation) of inner experience is a critical foundation for healing, but by itself, it's not enough. The Integral Recovery practitioner's witnessing capacity needs to be complemented and bolstered by specific techniques that deal with emotional upheaval and the integration of repressed material. Often we think that if we understand our issues, that somehow takes care of them. It doesn't. Understanding is nice, but it does not release, transform, and transmute our shadows and the repressed parts that are keeping us sick.

Both shadow work and the releasing of emotions are essential. I distinguish them in the following way: while shadow work deals with the content of repressed material, and uses any number of therapeutic techniques to uncover and integrate this material, releasing emotions deals with the emotional energy itself and trains the individual to simply release it or let it go, in the present moment. Classic examples of shadow work include psychoanalysis, gestalt therapy, and the "3-2-1 Shadow Process" taught by Ken Wilber and adapted by me for my work with Integral Recovery students.[1] Emotion work also comes in many varieties; I frequently use a technique taught by the Sedona Method.[2] This simple technique involves feeling the present emotion, asking oneself if one *could* release it, and then if one *would* release it, *when?* Even simpler is to say, on the in-breath, "I totally accept these feelings," and on the out-breath, "I release them." The content of the emotion is unimportant in this process. There is no need to get involved in self-analysis; rather, one simply feels the emotional energy (positive or negative) and practices welcoming it and letting it go. Letting it go does not mean pushing it out the door, but simply allowing the feeling to express itself in the body however it needs to. This can be done while sitting in meditation or at any time of day. Indeed, a practice of sitting meditation in conjunction with releasing emotions becomes the training ground for a moment-to-moment practice of releasing in the midst of everyday life.

This type of work is often referred to as mindfulness training. In this practice, one becomes mindful of, or gives attention to, a feeling without attempting to change, modify, or repress it. One simply observes it, allows the feeling to do what it needs to do, and then lets it go. The practitioner identifies with the awareness in which the emotion arises. This allows one to *disidentify* with the emotion or feeling, and in this greater spaciousness, the feeling or emotion naturally releases. As with all of our practices, this practice of mindfulness and emotional releasing becomes easier over time; it becomes second nature. In our IR work, this practice is especially essential, because early on some of the most powerful feelings that arise are cravings for drugs. The first time one confronts these cravings in early recovery can be very frightening, but with a few successful attempts at mindfulness, each subsequent experience of craving becomes easier to deal with. Psychologist Elisha Goldstein[3] calls this "riding the crave." Instead of being overwhelmed by the wave of cravings, one simply rides over it with the surfboard of mindfulness. The more experienced we become in dealing with our inner life and our emotions, the more we realize that negative feelings (cravings) are just feelings, and not the mortal adversaries we once thought they were.

Shadow Work

How do psychic fractures or dissociations (our shadows) play out in the catastrophic disease of addiction? As we said earlier, one of the main causes of chronic unrelieved stress, whose roots are deep within the unconscious, is unresolved trauma. Trauma is unresolved when the current self structure is not capable of absorbing or assimilating the overwhelming power of the trauma, or traumatic event, such as being sexually molested by one's father or seeing one's best friend's head blown off in combat. The magnitude and the power of these events are so strong that the psyche splits them off so that the self can survive. This is an amazingly effective survival strategy in terms of emotional first aid, but terribly harmful for long-term mental health. The unresolved traumas become split-off shadow elements that cause great suffering. These dissociated or repressed parts of us, these beasts in the basement of our consciousness, do not go to sleep but create absolute havoc in the pathological symptoms of depression, rage, self-hatred, hatred of others, anxiety, and chronic, inescapable stress. In the brain of the addict, the stress can manifest in triggering uncontrollable cravings for drugs, which is the disease of addiction. The very act of using these substances can be seen as an attempt to heal the suffering our split-off parts and repressed emotions produce.

As dependency on the substance(s) takes over, stress increases exponentially, and tolerance to the drug(s) becomes greater, resulting in increased consumption of more drugs that do less and less. The higher functions of the neocortex become progressively unplugged or become devoted to the reptilian brain stem's agenda: to scheme, scam, and get more drugs, whatever the price and no matter who gets hurt. Ken Wilber once said that the addict becomes "a walking reptilian brain stem." All of this is largely fueled by the inexorable power of the shadow.

Wilber often uses the following metaphor to explain the dynamics of the wounding, repressed shadow elements in our psyche that freeze up so much of our life energy and keep us stuck, unhealthy, and suffering. He explains it like this: When we are born, we have, say, $100 of life energy in our account. When we are small children and something bad happens, we lose $8. Then, as toddlers, some other unpleasant thing happens, and we repress the trauma, as it is too much to deal with at the time. This time, we lose another $10. This pattern keeps repeating itself until we are, say, 21 years old, and we are trying to make the transition into early adulthood that takes maybe a psychic minimum of $68. However, at that point, maybe we only have \$59 left in our energy account, and we just can't make the leap. Too much of our money has been lost in the shadows of the repressed parts of ourselves. Shadow work is the work of retrieving and reowning these split-off parts.

These split-off parts of ourselves can become independent subper-sonalities that exert tremendous control over our lives, becoming the source of personal failure, self-hatred, hatred of others, depression, and in the case of the addict, endless relapse. But if we go back, reown, and release these unresolved traumas and shadow elements, tremendous energy is released for growth, transformation, and creativity. This is what Carl Jung was referring to when he taught that God comes through our rejected parts.[4] There is tremendous energy frozen and locked up in these shadowy regions of disowned complexes. Therefore, if our adolescent, who is trying to get to young adulthood, goes back and releases these beasts in the basement, he now has \$98 back in his account instead of \$59, and he can accomplish the transition with vitality and health.

This powerful metaphor demonstrates why the emotional line is one of the essential lines included in Integral Recovery Practice. If one does not deal with these split-off objects or disowned subpersonalities, they will sabotage and limit healthy emotional growth and cause problems in other lines, which can lead to relapse after relapse, defeat, demoraliza-tion, and ultimately death, in the case of the addict. A point of tremen-dous importance in dealing with these split-off parts of ourselves is to remember that it is not enough to simply bring them into awareness, as in, "Oh, there you are!" Rather, they must be owned, felt, metabolized, and released. Otherwise, all sorts of unhealthy dissociative pathologies can develop. Failure to own, metabolize, and release/transform these shadow elements has had a large part, I believe, in the ineffectiveness of traditional treatment programs.

Freud said that the goal of analysis was "to make the unconscious conscious." Many decades of experience with therapists and their clients have shown that although bringing repressed material into conscious awareness is very interesting cognitively, and definitely explains a lot of dysfunction, it doesn't fix the problem. In fact, in many cases it makes the problem worse. Talk therapy alone often does more harm than good, as it can lessen the barriers to repression but then may cause the patient to be retraumatized, if she does not have a means for successfully deal-ing with the trauma.

The releasing process I teach generally begins like this: "While meditating, open into a relaxed state. Body relaxed, mind relaxed. Ask yourself, 'Is there anything that I need to learn or deal with that is getting in the way of my healing and happiness?' Sit with that, and see what arises. If nothing comes up, great, you're off the hook, so to speak. Enjoy the rest of your meditation. Our deep inner wisdom will bring up the material as we are ready, and as we invite it.

"If thoughts, memories, or sensations begin to arise, great! Don't force them; just watch with alertness and curiosity. If you feel sensations in your body, breathe into them and say in your mind, 'I welcome you, thank you for being here and showing up.' Remember these are disowned parts of your self, subpersonalities that are presenting themselves to be acknowledged, felt, and released."

There are several methods that we can employ to release the hurtful shadows. One is to acknowledge the feeling that has come up and watch it. On the in breath, say, "I welcome you," and on the out breath, "I release you." Continue this process while focusing on your heart area, or wherever sensations are being felt and intensified in the body. In doing this work, we are not only dealing with trauma and repressed unconscious material, we are also healing the body-mind split that so many of us suffer from, especially those of us who have suffered severe trauma in our past. (Many of us are cut off from our body and sensation.) Eckhart Tolle calls this the pain body, the place where our traumas and wounds congeal in our physical and subtle bodies. In our meditative practices, with our increasing awareness, this pain body arises clearly in our awareness where it then can be dealt with, healed, and released.

As we continue to master this practice, we notice a shift in our relationship to our body as our mind embraces it. This aids in establishing our physical and emotional health and promotes a new respect and trust in the wisdom that our bodies have for us. Our bodies do not lie. We may totally misinterpret the feelings and sensations that arise, but if we stay with the bodily felt sensations, own them, and allow them to release as they are ready, we will find that underneath those feelings, serenity and wisdom are available to us.

Remember, while doing this work, do not heed the thoughts that arise as the sensations intensify. These are the thoughts and stories that will keep you stuck. You do not have to repress them either, just bracket them, and continue to breathe into and release the completely owned and felt sensations. These memories and shadow aspects of ourselves are deeply embedded in our bodies. If we only deal with these feelings and emotions on an intellectual, cognitive basis, we are only halfway there, and the work is not complete.

Hale Dwoskin, teacher of the Sedona Method, a powerful method for healing one's emotional life, says, "If you are willing to welcome what you are experiencing in the moment, and at the same time choose to let go of the past responsibly, your emotional life gets richer and richer, and at the same time there is less and less attachment and aversion to that which is rising within you. You experience everything more fully." And, "Simply allow yourself to remain open inside, while your feelings come up and move through you. Look at each upset in your life as an opportunity for greater freedom . . . As you get into the habit of letting go in the moment as feelings arise, you'll develop a wonderful momentum that will support you when your deeper feelings surface. You will find it easier to let them go as well."[5]

For persistent issues more obviously related to our shadows, Ken Wilber and others have developed a process that he calls "The 3-2-1 Shadow Process." I have worked with this method and adapted it to the more specific needs of our Integral Recovery process. This process has proven itself a brilliant tool. As stated earlier, it is the split-off parts of ourselves, dwelling in the shadows of our psyche, that control us unconsciously and are a source of ongoing chronic stress that in the addict leads to powerful cravings, serial relapse, and the utter despair and demoralization that are the fate of the unhealed addict.

The 3-2-1 Shadow Process

> In this practice we begin the process of re-owning our shadow. We'll FACE our shadow in 3rd-person; we'll TALK to our shadow in a 2nd-person dialogue; and we'll BE our shadow in 1st-person. Face it, Talk to it, Be it . . . It's that simple.[6]

The parts of you that have been split off, dissociated, or repressed in your psyche manifest as symptoms: self-hatred, hatred of others, depression, self-destructive behaviors, destructive behaviors toward others or the environment, physical illness, and a myriad of other versions of these basic symptoms. In our depth meditation work, we invite these split-off parts of ourselves to show up and emerge (one at a time, please, otherwise it is too much). As a sub-personality emerges, we allow it to take a form in our imagination or mind's eye. Here, I will describe this process using an aspect of myself that looks like me, John, but many times people will see a dragon, a bear, an angry warrior, or some other symbolic representation of their dissociated personality.

When I do "3-2-1," I normally see a version of myself, for example, Rage-filled John, or Self-hating John, or whatever shadow aspect of myself is becoming conscious. So, for example, first I look at Self-hating John. I observe what he looks like. How is he holding his body? What are his facial expressions? What does the energy coming from his body feel like? This is the third-person perspective. You are looking at a part of yourself as if it were someone else. It is very important that you pay attention to any body sensations and feelings that come up as you do this, such as pain or constriction in the heart, belly or gut, in your throat, or even in your head behind your eyes. Normally, I find that about 60 percent of the time these feelings are centered in the heart chakra, but this is certainly not always the case, and attention and openness need to be brought to the place where these feelings are emerging.

Next, I begin a dialogue with myself, which is taking the second-person perspective. "Self-hating John, what are you feeling?" He says, "Self hatred!" And I ask, "Why do you feel that?" And he says, "Because I'm awful; I'm inadequate and cowardly . . ." or whatever the case may be. Then I ask Self-hating John, "Why do you feel this way?" And he will tell me. If you try this, you may be surprised to find that things are revealed to you that you were completely unaware of. In this case, Self-hating John usually reveals the history of the events or situations that gave rise to the self-hatred.

Be sure to pay attention to your bodily felt sensations throughout this process. It is very important to make sure that this work is anchored in the body for it to be complete and stick. Then I ask this part of myself, "What do you really need to be okay, Self-hating John?" He then tells me. "I need to forgive myself and know that I am loved," or whatever the case may be.

Once I get this second-person answer, this being the "2" of the 3-2-1 Shadow Process, I move into the first-person perspective and *become* Self-hating John. At this point, I am totally aware of what it is to be Self-hating John and feel all of his feelings in my body. I breathe in total acceptance and breathe out total release of these feelings of self-hatred, wherever I feel them in my body. You will know when the work is complete, as you will feel peace, spaciousness, and a new quality that has emerged; in the place of self-hatred there will be self-love and acceptance. This, in turn, can lead to a greater capacity to love and accept others for who they are.

This process is akin to the work of the alchemists of old. You actually transmute baser metals into gold, or, in our case, wounds, traumas, and shadow elements into healing positive qualities. New energy is added to our psychic bank accounts and is now available for transformation, growth, happiness, and creativity. Another great benefit from doing this work and practice is that as you continue your mastery of this skill, you can begin to release emotions even as they arise in the present. Say you are listening to the nightly news, and the information is so bleak and dark that you begin to feel despair or fear. Right in that moment, you can pay attention to your emotions and feelings, feel and invite them in completely, and then release them right away. Despair is then replaced by compassion, or some other quality that is a healthier response to what is occurring around you. In this way, you can keep yourself stress free, moment to moment, and not start a new process of creating and repressing shadow elements. This is a wonderful and, I believe, essential skill to master, as it leads us to greater wisdom and happiness. We are able to see all of the unpleasant negatives that arise in our lives and experience them not as "crap," but as fertilizer.

The same process can be done using positive feelings. You might think, "Why would I want to release a positive feeling?" Because beneath that positive feeling of getting the promotion, or winning the game, or being in love, lies something even better. As Integral scholar Sean Hargens[7] once told me, "I have learned that no matter what is going on, a part of me is always free."

Another method of dealing with emotions and shadow issues is one that I developed independently. It goes like this:

- identify the hurt in your body
- identify the thoughts associated with the hurt
- bracket or let go of the thoughts
- stay with the feeling in your body until it releases.

Remember, you don't have to do anything with the feeling—fix it, modify it, or repress it—just let the feeling do what it needs to do.

Finally, the simplest method of all, which is also effective, is feel it, bless it, and let it go.

Here is a wonderful poem by the thirteenth-century poet and mystic Rumi, in which he describes, in beautiful language, what we have been looking at.

The Guest House

This being human is a guest house.
Every morning a new arrival.
A joy, a depression, a meanness,
some momentary awareness comes
as an unexpected visitor.
Welcome and entertain them all!
Even if they're a crowd of sorrows,
who violently sweep your house
empty of its furniture,
still, treat each guest honorably.
He may be clearing you out
for some new delight.
The dark thought, the shame, the malice,
meet them at the door laughing,
and invite them in.
Be grateful for whoever comes,
because each has been sent
as a guide from beyond.[8]

That is it. If we open ourselves in our practice, each morning and throughout the day, these visitors will come—some pleasant, some awful, some terrifying. But come they will, and if we invite them in with gratitude, they will be our teachers and guides and will heal and revitalize our lives. If we do not invite them in, they will remain alive and well in our unconscious, where they will exert a powerful negative influence and control over our lives.

Note that sometimes these "guests" will stick around longer than we would like, and we may have to keep inviting a particularly powerful presence in to teach us. But know this: the greater the challenge, the greater the amount of transmuted energy is released in our lives for whatever is needed. Our psychic bank account fills up, and we have money to spare.

Trauma/shadow = opportunity for growth and transcendence, and the greater the trauma, the greater the opportunity.

At this point, I would like to quote a passage from *The Translucent Revolution*[9] by Arjuna Ardagh, which speaks to the issue of emotional release from the context of our expanded, larger self.

> As translucence deepens, our range of feeling, as well as our capacity to feel deeply, expands. We learn that it is possible to welcome grief, anger, even the depths of despair as waves, made of who we really are, and so as portals into a bigger love. Then feelings are more liquid, moving, flowing, and transforming continuously into one another, without the rigidity or charge of emotional drama. Feelings can exist as pure energy, without a story. Translucents have less resistance to feelings and embrace and welcome them as they arise. They discover how to feel into each one fully, to be complete with each experience rather than living in postponement. To the same degree that you have completely felt what is left from the past you can be total and present to meet life as it is in this moment.
>
> Translucents can access the limitless dimension of themselves with ease. At the same time, unlike our stereotypes of spiritual people, they make no attempt to renounce life. A translucent then, bridges the mystic and the enthusiastic participant, for when a translucent experiences feelings, even very painful ones, it is within the context of some connection to the limitless

This passage beautifully illustrates and clearly unpacks the practice and promise of Integral Recovery as it unites deep spiritual practice with deep emotional acceptance and releasing. I believe that it has been the very lack of a context or modality for deep emotional release and healing that has dogged our efforts at recovery for decades. Held within the context of the greater Self, which is quickly experienced in our deep meditative practices, traumatic feelings and negative emotions are no longer the enemy to be narcoticized or escaped from; instead they become our welcome teachers, providing us with energy and wisdom for growth, healing, and transformation. At this point, we can befriend our lives, our relations, our addictions, our past traumas, our shadows, and our emotions, because they are now held in a much greater context than we ever before imagined possible, and things begin to get very interesting.

It should be noted that not all repression involves repressing our negative aspects. There is also repression of the sublime. These locked up "light dragons" can be imagined, perhaps, in the attic, rather than in the basement, as they represent higher aspects of ourselves: our gifts, talents, and essentially our give-backs to life and to the world. There are vital things inside of us that long to be expressed and manifested. If we do not bring them forth, whether through sloth, fear, or negative self-opinion, they will fester inside of us and manifest as depression, cynicism, and jealousy (of others who brought forth their gifts). These positive repressions of our highest callings can cause as much illness, stress, and suffering as the negative repressions.

Jesus once said:

> If you bring forth what is within you,
> what you bring forth will save you.
> If you do not bring forth what is within you,
> what you do not bring forth will destroy you.

This is a quotation from the Gospel of Thomas, found near the Egyptian village of Nag Hammadi in 1945. I think this verse is deeply revealing regarding the necessity for service and creativity as essential emotional and spiritual needs for health and stable recovery. We need to access and bring out our gifts as a response to life, and in service to the times in which we find ourselves.

11

Healing the Spirit

Thus far, in the Integral Recovery model, I have covered the neurobiological basis for the disease of addiction, healing the body, transforming the brain, and healing the emotions. Now I am going to talk about healing your soul, or spirituality. This may be very interesting and attractive to some and repellent to others, depending on what your experience and history have been up to this point in your life. So, let us start by defining our terms. In Integral Recovery terms, spirituality deals with the most fundamental questions of life. Is there a God? Is there life after death? Is there a meaning and a purpose to life and the universe? Is there a personal purpose to my life that I must find? These are profound human questions, which confront us all, whether we choose to address them or not. They are a river we all have to cross, if we live long enough, and the purpose of this book, if you are an addict reading this, is to give you the opportunity to confront these questions.

Addressing the great existential questions of human existence involves looking beyond mere exteriors into the ground of being. It involves a profound inner journey, where we confront and, in some sense, overcome the sources of our dysfunction and suffering. This work can be framed in traditional religious terms or in secular ways. In the end, it probably doesn't matter. The quest itself is what produces the results.

I'm not going to give you easy answers or say things you must believe in order to be saved or recover, but I will tell you where to look to find answers for yourself, and I will share what I have found in my own looking and what others have reported. What you discover is your own and has to be if it is to have any profound and lasting value. As with all things Integral, your understanding of what you find will evolve and deepen as your practice continues. And let me say, too, that agnosticism and atheism are legitimate answers to the questions posed above. All I am asking is to keep an open mind and look in the direction in which I am pointing. If you already have a faith and a belief about such things, fine; what I am suggesting here will work for you in any case.

What I am suggesting is that you undergo a paradigm shift—not in the popular sense of a paradigm shift, in that you make up a new set of assumptions and beliefs about the nature of reality, but in the sense that you follow an injunction to practice using new techniques and technologies, which will provide you with new data that will shift and transform the way you understand reality.[1] The challenge, or injunction, as I present it in this Integral model, is *to look within*. The promise of spirituality is that when you do, you will find that your deepest self is your truest self and that this true self is what your heart and soul have always been seeking. As Mickey Gilley sang, "You've been looking for love in all the wrong places."

An important understanding that Integral Recovery brings to this spiritual practice, or injunction, is based on the work of Abraham Maslow, one of the great twentieth-century pioneers of both humanistic and transpersonal psychology. One of the many contributions that Maslow made was to observe that most of Western psychology up to that point had been based on the study of pathology, in other words, sick people. Maslow asked what would happen if we turned that on its ear and studied healthy people, really healthy people, to see if we could come up with any commonalities among them that we could learn from. Maslow proceeded to do just that and found a common denominator in these human exemplars or role models. He found that they all shared what he called a "peak experience." Sometimes it had only happened once, but in many cases it had happened more than once, if not often.

These peak experiences were characterized by intense, joyful feelings of peace and connectedness, and, in a very real but often mysterious way, a deep knowing that fundamentally things were okay, even if the observable data indicated otherwise. Now "peak" experience is just a secular, nonreligious way of saying "spiritual" experience. Maslow found that these peak experiences, or what are sometimes called "unitive" experiences, are necessary, almost like essential psychic nutrients, for a whole, healthy, and creative human being. Many of us have had these experiences in our lives already, facilitated by being in nature, music, making love, art, literature, seeing a newborn baby, and so on.

Many of us have also had peak experiences using mind-altering drugs, and it was the wonder of these experiences that led us to continue to use drugs. This resulted, however, not in liberation (maybe for a brief period) and higher growth, but in dependency, addiction, and eventually, total demoralization. For the addict, pursuing these types of experiences through drugs leads to a devastated life and a shameful death. Arrived at in the wrong way, these experiences are the equivalent of the sirens' song, which promises everything but leads to destruction. Come by in the right way, these experiences can be both useful and instructive, and cumulatively they can metabolize into energy and inspiration for higher stage growth.

Another aspect of Maslow's work, which we would do well to heed, is his hierarchy of needs.[2]

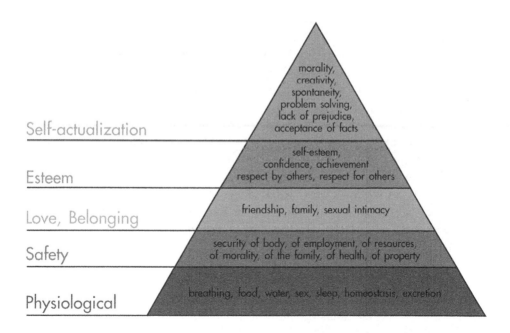

Figure 8. Maslow's Hierarchy of Needs Pyramid

As you can see from the illustration, the first rung in the ladder starts at very foundational stuff and works its way up from there, from survival to self-actualization needs. This is important, because as we have said before, the goal of Integral Recovery is not just ceasing to ingest addictive substances, but optimal health in all four quadrants, and sustained growth in your essential lines through an ongoing lifetime IRP. What this means is that once the lower rung needs are addressed and sufficiently satisfied, from the physiological to safety, from love and belonging to esteem, the question in life shifts radically from "What can I get?" to "What can I give?"

Some critics have pointed out, quite rightly, that this process is not as sequential as Maslow's model indicates. We can still be haunted by questions of higher meaning when our bills haven't been paid, there's no money in the bank, and the refrigerator is empty. However, it is also clear that there *are* depths of meaning beyond mere materialistic survival needs, and the capacity of people to address these deep, existential questions is greatly increased when the lower rung needs have been satisfied. (That is why the Lower-Right quadrant supports growth in the Upper-Left quadrant.)

The goal of Integral Recovery is to help our students skillfully repair and fulfill the lower-rung needs, and to prepare a strong foundation in all four quadrants so that the individual can more fully address the essential soul queries, "What can I give?" "How can I serve my people?" "Who are my people?" "What are my unique gifts that I am here to give?" "What kind of discipline and sacrifice will it take for me to do this?" When these questions arise, and they will as the Integral Recovery journey of healing and growth unfolds, you will be ready to embrace them and you will know you have come a long way from the narcissistic addict-self that lived by the creed that all that matters is "me" and getting high. I don't expect students in treatment to become Albert Schweitzers[4] in their first week of treatment and recovery, but be advised that this is the eventual high ground you are headed for, which will emerge from your practice and your healing process.

But, remember the old adage in the recovery world, "First things first." First, we create a safe environment for you away from the source and ability to get drugs and alcohol. Then we support you in detoxifying your body and restoring health and balance. At the same time, we establish emotional safety, and as the fog lifts and the mind begins to clear, we begin the work of transformation. In Integral Recovery terms, *transformation is positive change that lasts.*

Dr. Gary Nixon, a transpersonal psychologist on the faculty with the Addictions Counselling program at the University of Lethbridge, recently pointed out to me that addiction is "a counterfeit for the real quest for wholeness." If that is the case, and I think that it is, what, specifically, is addiction the counterfeit for? As I see it, there are three essential things that people are looking for when they begin to use drugs:

1. Escape from egoic suffering: By egoic, I do not mean selfish. Rather, I mean the suffering that is an inherent part of being a separate self in a human body. This suffering can be physical, emotional, or spiritual, and derive from any number of causes, but for all of us, suffering is an existential given. And drugs offer a very effective, if temporary, way out of that suffering. The problem is, of course, that as dependency takes over and use increases, the suffering is multiplied exponentially. Life becomes a literal "hell on earth."

2. Enhancement of pleasure: The desire to be more confident, more sensual, more intelligent, more creative, and so on. Again, there *is* often an experience of superior functioning, but it doesn't last. As the disease progresses, and the body, mind, and soul deteriorate, these temporary gains are lost.

3. Transcendence: One often experiences states of transcendence using mind-altering substances, where the body and the little mind are dropped temporarily, and one experiences a unitive state—a sense of expanded identity and consciousness. The problem is, as with all states, that they come and go. In the case of the drug user, this can often turn into a depressing letdown. Then one seeks the experience again and again through increased use of the drug, or trying new drugs or new combinations of drugs. But the experience never lasts, and it is never quite as good as the first time. This is called "chasing the high" and is a downward spiral to insanity, addiction, and death.

The good news is that the quest for these qualities is not bad; in fact, it is dead on. I believe these drives are essential to realizing our highest aspirations as human beings; only the method is at fault, in this case drugs. Legitimate ways of achieving these goals involve practice. The recovering addict must learn that these goals are indeed legitimate and are achievable in ways that are a thousand times better than their counterfeit counterparts. It is essential for recovery that students realize this and begin to experience this very early on. If the choice is between addiction and depression, addiction will win almost every time.

Spirituality is one of the essential lines we work with on our journey toward transformation, sobriety, and optimal health, because without a vital spiritual connection and the light and liberation it brings to our goal of Integral health, sobriety will not happen. The spiritual meditative experiences that we encounter in our daily practices actually have transformative effects in our healing ability, sobriety, and health. These experiences are not just fascinating and cool (which they definitely are) but are also an essential part of our ongoing healing and transformative process. The mystics have always known this, and science is beginning to understand this. Let me emphasize, this is probably not the spirituality that you have heard about in church or that you hear preachers preaching about on TV and on the radio. I am talking about using the eye of deep introspection to relax into your body and to relax into your thoughts and emotions in a systematic daily practice, aided by teachers who have themselves taken the plunge into their deepest selves. It is about committing to this process with heroic intent and singleness of purpose, which will allow you to achieve the results you are looking for.

Until One is Committed[5]

Until one is committed, there is hesitancy, the chance to draw back, always ineffectiveness. Concerning all acts of initiative (and creation) there is one elementary truth, the ignorance of which kills countless ideas and splendid plans: that the moment that one definitely commits oneself, then Providence moves too. All sorts of things occur to help one that would never otherwise have occurred. A whole stream of events issues from the decision, raising in one's favor all manner of unforeseen incidents and meetings and material assistance, which no man could have dreamed could have come his way.

—William Hutchinson Murray

In Sanskrit, there is the phrase "neti, neti," which means "not this, not this." It well describes the first stage in meditation, when we no longer identify with the objects of our consciousness, such as thoughts, feelings, emotions, body, world, and so on. In developing a meditative practice, we learn to identify with our higher context (or Higher Power) as opposed to our content (the objects that arise in thought); we identify with being the paper instead of the words on the paper; or with being the sky itself and not the clouds; or with the pure Transcendent Witness or consciousness versus the "things" that arise in consciousness. These moments of translucence, when the relative passing world is penetrated by the light of the eternal, can become moments of profound healing and reordering of our lives, and their effect spills out beyond the meditative hour to flavor and influence every aspect of our lives. This is why a profound, ongoing, contemplative, meditative practice is essential to Integral Recovery.

Let us listen to the words of the great Catholic monk and mystic Thomas Merton:

> From the viewpoint of our separate self
> and smaller will,
> it's normal to act on the basis
> of our own desires and preferences;
> when we surrender our smaller self and will
> to the guidance of a higher will
> and dedicate our actions
> for the highest good of all concerned,
> we feel an inspired glow
> at the center of our life.

And again.

> Life is this simple:
> We are living in a transparent world,
> and God shines through in every moment.
> This is not just a fable or a nice story;
> it is living truth.
> If we remember God, abandon ourselves to God,
> and forget ourselves,
> we may see this truth:
> God manifests everywhere, in everything.
> We cannot be without God.
> It's impossible.
> It's simply impossible.

What Merton is describing here are the spiritual qualities that begin to emerge from a deep and sustained meditative practice. Even though Merton speaks from within the Christian tradition, his concepts are universal.

The Transformational Event

Traditionally, in AA terminology the transformative event that leads to the willingness to do the necessary work is called "hitting bottom." This is when the shame, failure, and suffering caused by using drugs are simply no longer options or acceptable to the addict. The precipitating transformational motivators often come in the form of lost jobs, changed locks, criminal charges, and jail time. Bill Wilson described this as the utter deflation and demoralization that were the precipitating factors that led to his spiritual awakening and eventually to the creation of Alcoholics Anonymous. In many cases, if not most of the time, the motivators are of an external nature: the intervention of family, friends, the law, or bosses simply leaves the suffering addict no wiggle room, and this leads to surrender and acceptance. "Okay, what do I have to do?"

While Bill Wilson was in the hospital dying from alcoholism (around the same time that his spiritual awakening occurred, after which he never drank again), he came across the book *The Varieties of Religious Experience*, by William James. In this classic volume on psychology of spiritual experience, James says that powerful transformational experiences are often preceded by a powerful ego deflation, or what is called in spiritual circles a "dark night of the soul" (St. John of the Cross).

At the point of deepest despair, the light breaks through, and it is the dawn of a new day and a new level of depth and understanding. This dark night is the transformational chaos that allows the next higher order to emerge. This is why many recovering addicts whom I have known speak of their disease of addiction as their greatest gift and blessing, because it set the groundwork and conditions for their eventual recovery and transformation. The dark energy of addictive suffering becomes the negative entropy of spiritual emergence and renewal.

Very interestingly, we find that as we continue our Integral Recovery Practice, we experience new dark nights that are part and parcel of the ongoing journey of awakening and transformation. This is not a one-time deal, but as we achieve mastery, we can welcome and work with these chaotic dark spots on our journey and actually bless them as they arise, for we know that chaos is truly the mother of our individual and collective evolution.

One of the great wisdoms of Bill Wilson and Alcoholics Anonymous was Bill's willingness to allow members of AA to connect with "a God of their own understanding." Bill Wilson came from a Christian tradition; in fact, he took many of the principles of AA from a Christian Evangelical organization known as the Oxford Group.[6] Bill could have easily gone with the line that in order to become sober you must receive Jesus as your Lord and Savior, but he did not. He was not about saving souls, but getting people sober, and he realized early on that it was important not to alienate anyone, so he made the only necessity for membership in AA "a desire for sobriety."

Building on this tradition in Integral Recovery, we do not push any brand of religion or tradition. Instead we give our students the tools to begin their own journeys to the center of their beings. What they find at their deepest levels is just what they find. They may return from this journey a Christian, a Jew, a Moslem, a pagan, an agnostic, a Buddhist, or something else, but what they *will* encounter is a great mystery that answers the deepest longing of their hearts.

Step Eleven of the Twelve Steps of AA reads, "Sought through prayer and meditation to improve our conscious contact with God as we understood him." Time after time, I have heard from those who have successfully maintained their sobriety through AA that spirituality was the key. I also noted that generally AA did not avail itself of the tremendous reservoirs of contemplative wisdom both from the East and from the West; there was precious little information or injunctions on how one should conduct a meditative practice, maybe the most important of the steps. Most of what is presented in the *Big Book* of Alcoholics Anonymous are formulaic, petitionary prayers such as St. Francis' prayer, "Lord make me an instrument of your peace . . ." The prayers contained in the *Big Book* are wonderful and very noble, but they are not a substitute for a contemplative/meditative practice (although I have used the St. Francis prayer for years in my own inner work).

An extraordinary aspect of Integral Recovery is that deep spiritual experiences become the personal realizations of all those who do the practices, that do the injunctions. Spiritual realizations are no longer just the purview of the spiritual elite or the masters in any given tradition, but of every one of us; they are our human birthright, now achievable by the many. Let us listen once more to Arjuna Ardagh as he describes the "radical awakening" so many people are now experiencing, which I believe is the way out of the trance of addiction.

We call such a shift in awareness a "radical awakening." It is the
moment when you taste reality outside the limiting confines
of the mind, the body, beyond birth and death, eternally free.
Despite the activity of thought and feeling, you know yourself to be the silence experiencing that movement. It is the
moment when you intuit the real potential of life, free from
the incessant mental machinery of complaint and ambition. A
radical awakening often releases a tidal wave of creativity and
generosity of spirit, a natural impulse to serve and contribute.
In these moments, we know that love is who we are, not
something we sometimes feel.[7]

The 1-2-3 of God

Earlier, in chapter 10, on healing emotions, I related the 3-2-1 Shadow
Process, which is the ability to take a first-, second-, and third-person
perspective on our shadow material. In a similar vein, we also have what
is called the 1-2-3 of God, based on the work of Ken Wilber. What this
process allows us to do is take different first-, second-, and third-person
perspectives in our spiritual practices as well. Let me explain.

In our spiritual practice, when we are in meditation or prayer, as
the case might be, there are three basic perspectives that we can take
on divinity, God, or spirit. The third perspective, "3," or third person, is
the perspective we take in our contemplation or meditation when we
think of spirit as something objective, something out there or up there,
as when we might say, "Isn't God wonderful," or, "Isn't God a bummer."
Here we are speaking of God as being something other than ourselves
or the people we are conversing with. For example, we might experience
this when we look at the night sky in Southern Utah and feel absolutely
humbled and in awe of the beauty that confronts us. "Wow, the universe
is so amazing!" Or, "Isn't creation so incredible." This is a third-person
perspective: "I'm not talking to the universe; I'm not feeling like I am
the universe; I am talking about the universe."

In the second-person relationship with spirit or God, I am actually talking to divinity as an other that I am in relationship with, as in,
"God, I love you," or, "Lord, show me your will." And, a first-person
relationship with God or spirit consists of those moments when the
boundaries between our ego selves, our small selves, and God dissolve

and there is no "other"; there is simply I AM. As Integral practitioners, we know that if we neglect any of these perspectives, then we have left out a perspective that is actually essential, thereby impoverishing our spiritual practice.

One of the problems that often happens in spiritual development, after people advance from a blue/mythic fundamentalist stage of spirituality, is that they tend to believe that any second-person relationship with the divine is somehow superstitious or juvenile, and they leave it behind. Often, because people equate religion or spirituality with fundamentalism, they leave religion or spirituality behind altogether. Ken Wilber refers to this as a level/line fallacy. This is where people believe that all religion or spirituality is blue fundamentalist hogwash and can't be taken any further.

The truth is that spirituality is not only expressed in blue fundamentalist terms, but continues all the way up our spiral of human development. Therefore, there is a blue version of spirituality, and an orange, green, second-tier, and third-tier version. As Rollie Stanich, a teacher of Integral Christianity, says, "We see God through colored glasses." So, what I am saying with the 1-2-3 of God is that we no longer have to equate second-person relationship with God as an anachronism that must be left behind as we move from blue to higher stages of development. We can maintain and honor and grow with a second-person perspective all the way up the spiral. Try it; I think you'll like it.

The first-person, the "1" of God, includes those moments in meditation or prayer when the boundaries between ourselves and spirit, or God as "other," dissolve. Then there is no longer me and you, there is only I AM. The very fact that Integral theory even makes us aware that we have the option of taking these perspectives in our spiritual practice allows us to deepen and enrich our inner life.

Just as many folks moving beyond blue have a problem with a second-person perspective or relationship to the divine, so also do many blue-level spiritual practitioners have a problem with a first-person perspective, where God is no longer other, and there is only I AM. The fear is, it seems, that you will begin to believe that you are God! Which is true, in a nondual, ultimate sense, but this doesn't mean that your small ego, all your hatreds and foibles and loves and cravings and desires, and so on, is God in the sense that it created and runs the universe. Sorry, it just ain't so. To believe otherwise is simply a case of misbegotten narcissism. There are not too many problems with the third-person perspective, unless you are an atheist and get annoyed with God talk at all. But even an atheist can talk about the history of religion or the history of God, such as in Karen Armstrong's excellent book, *A History of God*.[8]

A second-person relationship to the divine is one of the gifts of an Integral approach to spirituality, elucidated by Wilber in his book *Integral Spirituality*.[9] Many of us, when we grow beyond the mythic, absolutistic stage of blue, lose this sense of intimacy and our one-to-one relation with Spirit. We think it is childish and/or superstitious. Wilber has shown how we can re-own this relationship to the divine. Not only can we re-own it, but if we don't, we impoverish ourselves by leaving out this perspective. This is good news to all you closet lovers of God. And for those of you who have never experienced this sort of relation with Spirit, give it a shot. The literature is ancient, rich, and deep that describes this sacred relationship to Spirit as Other. Using this perspective in our spiritual practice deepens the quality of our inner work.

A time-honored method of establishing a second-person relationship to the divine is simply praying to your Higher Power, asking for a pure heart and good motives. As Jesus beautifully put it in the Sermon on the Mount, "Blessed are the pure in heart for they shall see God." I would like to include the prayer I have used for years in my contemplative practice, the Prayer of St. Francis.[10] This prayer is so right-on and powerful that it has been used and adopted by many other traditions besides Christianity. Note also, when one practices visualizations, affirmations, or prayers, in the very deep brainwave states facilitated by brainwave entrainment technology, they become deeply imprinted into your unconscious mind. They are thus enabled to help heal, purify, and focus the power of the unconscious, in ways we are just beginning to understand. I would like to quote the prayer in its entirety here, because of its beauty and power as a contemplative tool, but also in homage to Bill Wilson and the *Big Book* of AA, who also quote this great prayer.

> Lord, make me an instrument of Thy peace.
> Where there is hatred, let me sow love;
> where there is injury, pardon;
> where there is doubt, faith;
> where there is despair, hope;
> where there is darkness, light;
> and where there is sadness, joy.
>
> O Divine Master, grant that I may not so much seek
> to be consoled as to console;

to be understood, as to understand;
to be loved, as to love.
For it is in giving that we receive;
it is in pardoning that we are pardoned;
and it is in dying that we are born to Eternal Life.
Amen.[11]

Four Essentials for Integral Spiritual Practice

What distinguishes our Integral approach to spirituality and the spiritual line are the following four aspects that must be included, comprehended, and used. They, I believe, distinguish Integral spirituality, and hence Integral Recovery, from any other approach that is currently being used, whether premodern, modern, or even postmodern.

The first aspect that must be included is what I call "essence." We must have a spiritual practice that allows us to experience our deepest nature or true self. This will be referred to in many different ways, according to one's level or tradition (or nontradition). This essence might be referred to variously as spirit, God, emptiness, Original Face, true nature, or so on. In order for our spiritual practice to be based on something more than blind faith or dogma, in other words, believing what some other person says about his experience of the ultimate, we must have a practice that allows us to voyage into this territory ourselves. This is the area that is often referred to, in mystical or Integral parlance, as the nondual, or the first-person perspective of the divine. At this essential or deepest level of reality, our ego boundaries and separateness dissolve. We realize experientially that there is truly only One and that we are it and always have been. This is often referred to as Self-realization, or a mystical, unitive experience of God. In this experience, the realization is of the big Self, that beyond our ego, individuality, and history. We are That, the I AM that is spoken of in the book of Genesis.

I have found that in my own practice, and in my work with my students, these states of consciousness and realizations, however fleeting, begin to come online quite quickly using our Integral maps and our brainwave entrainment enhanced meditation techniques. This is when we realize that we are the pure emptiness or pure awareness from which everything, including our own bodies and egos, arises, moment to moment. As we go through our own internal archeological digs in our meditations, through layer after layer of our histories, woundings, memories, experiences, and so on, we come to a vast ocean of stillness, which is often referred to in Buddhist speak as Emptiness. This is not to be confused with nothingness, as in Western existential thought. This emptiness might be referred to as the Creative Void or the Matrix that everything arises from; immersion in which produces bliss, compassion, and wisdom.

So for a spiritual practice to be Integral, it must allow for this nondual realization of our deepest self. And, not only must it awaken us temporarily, as in, "Dude, I remember taking mushrooms in Oxaca in 'sixty-eight . . . wow!" but it must keep us awake and deepen that awakening. As Ken Wilber is wont to quote Zen master Roshi Baker, "Enlightenment is an accident, but practice makes us accident prone."

The second essential aspect for an Integral Spiritual Practice is adding the developmental spiral to our conception of spirituality and recovery. This provides a quantum leap in our understanding of the evolutionary process of recovery and becoming the highest and best version of ourselves, as well as a hugely useful map to chart our own individual progress. It goes a long way to explaining why devout religionists are often knocking heads in their interpretations and understanding of ultimate truth. One thing we are learning is that sustained Integral practice makes our evolutionary journey up the spiral of development happen more quickly and healthily in that the growth is not unbalanced. One of Ken Wilber's great insights into this developmental journey is that when certain lines are left behind, such as the emotional line, severe pathologies can develop, despite high spiritual understanding and realization even into second and third tier.

I have worked with students who, when they have begun to sober up, were fully green in the ethical line in their holistic, nonjudgmental, compassionate ideals; however, because of unresolved trauma in the emotional line, they were, at the same time, narcissistic, self-absorbed, and emotionally very immature. So, again, if the four essential self-related lines that we work with in our IRP—body, mind, heart, and spirit—are not close in their developmental level, pathologies do occur, which can eventually or quite quickly lead to relapse, collapse, and even death in the case of our addicts. By knowing this, we can prescribe extra work and care to the inferior and undeveloped aspects. In the case of the narcissistic, self-absorbed, and immature, there are a number of practices such as therapy, service-oriented work, and shadow and trauma work that can be used to strengthen and elevate this pathologically low line.

The third essential aspect is states of consciousness. As we have said before, there are certain basic states in a normal 24-hour period, such as waking and dreamless sleep, but states also include all the emotions and feelings that arise moment to moment in our lives, whether they are joy, depression, love, hate, despair, boredom, or curiosity. Remember, states are the clouds in the sky, the birds, the airplanes, and the bugs, that arise in the vastness of our own being. With this knowledge and practice, we can learn to release our negative emotions and no longer be their slaves. This also includes traumas and buried issues from our past. How do we do this? The simplest explanation is radical acceptance. We absolutely open to and allow whatever state of consciousness is arising in our awareness, without judgment, and without following the mental obsessive thoughts and chatter that accompany these states. We simply stay with the states as they express themselves in our awareness and our bodies. In this way, they pass quickly and can be welcomed as teachers and allies in our process of living and being fully awake. We learn that all these states are not ultimate in their nature; they come and go and arise in that which is ultimately our true nature or pure consciousness.

By radically surrendering and not trying to "fix," medicate, stuff, avoid, or project unpleasant states that arise, we become free. We understand that absolutely nothing can destroy our true nature or the wisdom and equanimity that come with this understanding of, and identification with, our deepest, truest self.

The fourth and last, but not by any means least, essential aspect is the shadow. Again, I deeply bow to the great wisdom of Ken Wilber in including the shadow as an essential aspect of the Integral map. Without the key of the shadow, all our work is done in vain; our spiritual communities become cults, our teachers become tyrants, our recoveries are temporary, our hope is forlorn, and our future on this planet is devolutionary and catastrophic.

In the shadow, in these unconscious parts of ourselves that are truly the bottom of the iceberg, there abides great energy and power. If these shadow parts of ourselves are left locked or medicated into unconsciousness, they will destroy us. That which is locked in the basement will grow in the front yard and not only grow, but grow into something terrible and destructive. These shadow regions of our psyche hide not only our negative aspects, but also our greatest gifts and talents. Positive or negative aspects of ourselves, left in the unconscious and unattended to, will cause destructive pathologies as we either hurt ourselves or die of despair from never knowing our unrealized potentials, causing the world around us to wither from our ungiven gifts.

In so many of our religions and myths, it is clearly recognized that the hero's journey must, and I say again, *must*, include a descent into the underworld and the facing of our dragons, our own mortality, our fears, and death, in order for rebirth and resurrection to happen. The journey to God, as Franciscan priest Richard Rohr so clearly teaches, is through the darkness. These unrealized, unresolved, unhealed, and unilluminated parts of ourselves, if left in the shadow or the unconscious, will defeat us and eventually kill us, both individually and collectively. However, brought to light, owned, transmuted, and included, these shadow elements, both individual and collective, become a source of unbelievable creative energy that gives us the capacity to have compassion, love deeply, and creatively and beautifully participate in the evolutionary unfolding of our time.

So, for our spiritual practice and work to be truly Integral and comprehensive, these four columns of the temple must be included. Again, these are not merely intellectual understandings but must be fully embodied and incorporated parts of our living Integral practice.

Practice and the Path to Mastery

Mastery, and recovery, means staying on the path. Every day you may make progress. Every step may be fruitful. Yet there will stretch out before you an ever-lengthening, ever-ascending, ever-improving path. You know you will never get to the end of the journey. But this, so far from discouraging, only adds to the joy and glory of the climb.

—Sir Winston Churchill

If people knew how hard I worked to get my mastery, it wouldn't seem so wonderful after all.

—Michelangelo

If AQAL is the map that illumines the journey, then our Integral Recovery Practice becomes the landscape itself. It bears repeating, and repeating often, because of the centrality of this crucial point: Integral Recovery is a lifelong practice that is the journey to self-mastery. It is characterized by what evolutionary scientists call "punctuated equilibrium." In other words, we make dramatic transformational leaps forward, separated by relatively long plateau periods, punctuated by powerful transformational leaps to yet higher levels of development. It is important to understand the dynamics of mastery and apply them to our Integral Recovery practices so that we do not become attached (addicted) to the transformational climaxes themselves. This would be only another addictive pattern and lead to failure when expectations are not met.

Understanding that every practice is inevitably characterized by a series of plateaus that are punctuated by bursts of progress is essential for a successful recovery. I first noted the "plateaus then progress" phenomenon while I was studying German at the Defense Language Institute (DLI).

DLI was probably the premier language school in the world at the time, where the military taught and fulfilled its need for linguists. The teaching was very intense, and there was a large dropout rate. (Those familiar with German grammar can sympathize with the difficulty of my task.) A pattern that has since become familiar to me in other areas of study and practice is that I go for a while, not feeling that I am getting anywhere, and then suddenly I kick into a new level of fluency or capacity. All at once, things reorganize or reconstellate in my head, and, in this case, I abruptly started to understand and speak German at a level of proficiency that I had not thought possible. I noticed this pattern with German over and over; and the same thing occurred with my guitar playing, tennis, strength training, and so on.

Most of the time, we work at our current stage development. Wilber calls this "translation," which means we are doing the work of balancing all four quadrants at the stage or structure that we currently call home. This work, of course, is setting the stage for vertical growth to the next stage, which we call transformation. Any deficiencies in our horizontal work will make for problems and pathologies in our next emergent stage.

In a talk I attended recently with Zen teacher Diane Musho Hamilton, she stated that there were five reasons to practice meditation, in this case Zen meditation:

1. For all the physiological benefits of meditation: improved bio-balance in the body and brain, stress reduction, lower blood pressure, etc. (The stuff that is highlighted in the popular press about meditation and its health benefits.)

2. To increase mental focus

3. Self-realization, or as Zen practitioners describe it, "remembering your Original Face"

4. To increase compassion—that is, to break down the walls and structures that keep our species at odds with itself

5. And last, because that is what buddhas (awakened ones) do. We practice because it is an expression of life's drive to self-transcendence. We practice because of what we are and to become what we will be. Thus, we unite in our practice emptiness and form, being and becoming, the eternal and the evolutionary.

All of these reasons to practice apply equally well to our Integral Recovery work. When our Integral Recovery Practice becomes so central to our being that there is no goal, when the goal and the journey are one, we are entering the zone of the nondual. Here, there is no tension between being and becoming; there is only the eternal I AM that is the dynamic and thrusting forward power of the evolving universe as well as the eternal presence of stillness and pure awareness that is our deepest and truest Self.

It is important not to see IR as a quick fix, but as a reordering of our understanding of life and how life itself is to be practiced, as a practice. There is nothing wrong with enjoying the fruits of an IRP, feeling better in our bodies, getting free of the past, increased intelligence, creativity, and so on, but what keeps us going? At the plateau times, it is the intrinsic joys of practice itself.

Much has recently been written about the science of practice, transformation, and indeed the creation of genius and extraordinary abilities.[1] We have been living with the old cultural story that some of us are just born with "it" for a long time. Genius, that is. They are "naturals." Individuals such as Mozart, Ted Williams, Jimi Hendrix, and others have been used to bolster this idea of born geniuses. Well, apparently we got it wrong. Geniuses are not born; they are made. People of extraordinary ability and talent are crafted and honed in the fires of persistent, dedicated, deep, and deliberate practice. Several recent books, such as *The Talent Code*, *Talent Is Overrated*, *Living Deeply: The Art and Science of Transformation in Everyday Life*, and *The Genius in All of Us* are pointing out a new story in which extraordinary abilities are created—not given—which puts us completely back on the hook of responsibility for achieving our highest abilities and our greatest calling. Again and again, when we begin to look into our cultural assumptions of being born a genius or a "natural," we find another story emerging.

The young Mozart did not write musical masterpieces, but he did have an extraordinary music teacher in his father. Mozart's early musical works were quite repetitive and unoriginal in their structures. It was not until later in life that Mozart created his true masterpieces. This was after having written hundreds, if not thousands, of musical pieces and scores prior to his breakthroughs. The young Mozart was brilliantly trained by his father and exhibited a profound curiosity and passion for learning. And again, Ted Williams' perfect swing was crafted from his childhood with hours and hours and hours of practice on his own or with the help of his young friends.

In a study at a top English academy of music,[2] the questions posed were, What causes greatness in the students? What is the difference between the top students, those who are assured of going on to have careers as soloists on the stages of the world; students who will become journeymen, instrumentalists, and third or fourth chairs in orchestras; and the marginal students who are barely keeping up in school and who will most likely fail. The one constant, found across the spectrum from the very good students to the average and the mediocre, was the amount of time spent practicing daily. It was not economic, it wasn't ethnic, and it wasn't even students' IQ scores. On average, the master students practiced 2 hours a day, the average students practiced an average of 45 minutes a day, and the poor students practiced an average of 15 minutes a day.

Researchers also looked at the question, If practice is the key to greatness in any particular activity (or line), then what characterizes this transformative practice, and why do some people do the hard work and others not. Deep and deliberate practice, as it has been characterized, is often not fun and can be challenging, difficult, and sometimes even boring. So, how does this happen? More often than not, researchers found that there is an initiatory experience, such as the young Eric Clapton had upon hearing an old blues record on the radio, or some experience that acts as an attractor and inflames the imagination of the future master.

Many times there is a skillful mentor or coach who helps the young student, in the early days, on his path to mastery. (This is often my work—that of coach and mentor to my clients in the early days of their IR treatment.) After the initial phase, the practice and the practitioner take on a life of their own. There is an intrinsic joy to practice, and the better one gets, the deeper the particular activity becomes; it begins to reveal itself as a field of almost infinite learning and discovery.

Now, if you are reading this and thinking, "Oh, I am old, and I never had a flash bang experience like Eric Clapton, and I don't and never did have a great mentor and teacher," the good news is that most extraordinary achievers were and are late bloomers. Most often, child prodigies do not blossom into great achievers as adults. They seem to do pretty well in general, but on average they don't achieve great things as adults.

The theory is that this happens because they are rewarded for their particular gifts and then don't have much motivation to push beyond that ability. A test was done with two groups of students,[3] who, after they had performed a particular activity, were told either, "You're really smart at that" or "You must have worked really hard to be able to do that." Later, when the two groups were given new and challenging tasks to perform, the ones that had been praised for their hard work were eager to get on with the new challenge, and those who had been praised for their natural ability and smartness were not. What happens in adult great achievers is that they come to the realization that the process of self-improvement is in their own control.

Let me also give you a historical example. Winston Churchill, who almost everyone would agree was a great achiever, who virtually held out alone to keep the British in the fight against the Nazi empire, perhaps saved the Western world as we know it and perhaps preserved political freedom in the world for generations to come. He was also, by the way, awarded the Nobel Prize for Literature[4] and authored more than 70 books. Yet Churchill was anything but a child prodigy. In fact, his father, Randolph Churchill, considered him to be slow and with very little potential.

Winston's early educational experience was poor, and he had to take the test to enter the Royal Military Academy Sandhurst three times before he passed. Sandhurst, the British equivalent of West Point,[5] was often a place reserved for the less talented and gifted members of the English aristocracy during the Victorian era. Winston did all right at Sandhurst and achieved renown on the polo field, as he was an excellent horseman. But it was not until he arrived at his first duty station in India that he began a radical program of self-education and self-improvement. He read volumes of philosophy, science, and history and wrote extensive papers and essays on the subjects he was studying. During this period, he also began to sharpen his skill in writing and using the English language.

What motivated Winston were probably several things, including, perhaps, a desire to show his father that he was wrong. But, chiefly what causes someone to work this hard on self-improvement is what is called "a rage for mastery."[6] Winston realized that he could improve himself and his abilities and soon began to supplement his meager military wages with good money from the articles he was writing. Years later, Winston became not only a Nobel Prize–winning author, but also a world-famous orator, with an amazing capacity to use the English language and inspire millions of his countrymen and Americans during England's "darkest hours."

Another interesting note to this is that Winston's famous oratory skills were not natural. In fact, he stuttered and had a speech impediment. Winston would spend literally hours practicing a speech he was going to give to the House of Commons in front of a mirror, working on his gestures, intonations, and words to such a degree that his speeches would literally captivate the House of Commons and inspire even those who did not agree with him politically. His voice of courage, resistance, and tenaciousness under the threat of the Nazi empire inspired the world and most probably changed the course of history.

Thinking back on my own more than 40 years of playing the guitar, I am amazed that I was able to get past the stage when it took much effort to form, say, a D chord on the neck of my guitar. But I had a driving passion and a good teacher—my best friend, Buzzy Denham. Did I have a moment like Eric Clapton that woke me up to the beauty of the guitar? I can't remember specifically, but I know my generation, coming of age in the sixties and early seventies, was steeped in the music of the times. I never wanted music to be merely a spectator activity; I wanted to participate and feel the music coming through my fingers, my body, my soul, my Self.

I did reach a high level of proficiency as a rhythm guitarist, singer, and songwriter and have played and recorded for decades now. More recently, and I believe this is largely because of my own Integral practice, I hit another one of those great leaps forward and have again taken up the practice of playing the guitar, in this case the electric blues guitar. It seems to me I have tapped into a mystery of almost infinite depth of beauty. This, after figuring, in my late forties, that I had gotten about as good as I was going to get with the guitar.

Let me say this: Practice is not just going to a gym and chatting with your neighbors or plunking around on the guitar idly for a few minutes. It means deep and deliberate repetitive daily work, in which one pushes oneself beyond one's comfort zone to the place of discomfort and failure. If you want to get stronger, you have to push your body beyond what it can easily do; if you want to grow as a guitarist or an instrumentalist, you have to work on riffs, scales, and rhythms that seem beyond your capacity. And with concentration, focus, and repetitive determination, one can almost feel the new neural pathways that are forming in the brain and the new capabilities that are arising out of the creative chaos of deep practice and in the pushing of ourselves beyond whatever we believed we could do. Over time, through the ups and downs, the plateaus and the leaps forward, we gain confidence in the practice of practice itself, and our self-created boundaries about who we are and what the limits of our capacities are begin to dissolve and extend into a future that we can sense but cannot yet clearly see. What is creative is truly novel, and we just can't know what that next stage is going to feel like and produce through us.

Science is now revealing what the history of our great artists, thinkers, and achievers has always revealed, namely, that there is a way to greatness, growth, and transcendence. And that is practice, practice that continues over thousands of hours and through years of dedicated concentration. It isn't easy. It's hard, sometimes monotonous, and even discouraging. But ultimately it is glorious and life affirming. In my own mind, I sometimes call it the Gospel, or the Good News, of practice. This is again confirmed by the latest cutting-edge findings of neuroscience as to the absolute plasticity of the human brain, its ability to evolve, heal, and grow at whatever stage of development, with the appropriate support, techniques, and technologies. It is also confirmed in the growing science of epigenetics, which shows us that our genetic makeup is the smallest factor in determining who or what we become. It shows us that genetics x environment = ability or talent.

For example, I have on my desk as I write this a beautiful and extremely powerful computer that is connected to millions and millions of people around the world through the internet. (As of this writing, 2,095,006,005 people are connected to the internet according to InternetWorldStats.com.) The hardware, and in some sense the software, of this computer is equivalent to my genetic makeup. However, what I can do with this computer has almost infinite possibilities—among them the creation of masterpieces of literature, mathematics, science, poetry, art, film, and relationships—again limited only by my skill, determination, and imagination.

It has been said by Wilber and other social historians[7] that modernity began with the discovery of evolution. In other words, that we and life itself started out as very simple processes and then, over a very short cosmological period of time, became very complex and ever more conscious and capable. We are the products of evolution, modernity told us. Perhaps in the next stage that is bursting forth, the postpostmodern world, we are coming to understand that not only are we the products of an evolutionary process, but we also can become the conscious and responsible instruments of our evolutionary desires and growth. Think about this for a moment. If we would show up for ourselves, for our families, for our world, roll up our sleeves, and dedicate ourselves to the process of our own healing and transformation, cultivating our wisdom, compassion, and abilities, there is no end in sight to this journey that we have embarked upon. We simply do not know the limits of our own capacities and potential for achievement, compassion, and connection. The only way we can fail in our humanity, or in our recovery, is if we do not take up the task and challenge of mastery, through informed, skillful practice dedicated to the essential evolutionary parts of us and to the talents and gifts that our souls tell us we are here to bring into the world.

In Integral Recovery, our practices facilitate a new inner vision—one that allows us to construct an innovative, deeply realized, and transformed image of ourselves and our place in the universe. This new paradigm is characterized by lives that are deeply impregnated with meaning, love, and connection, and a fresh sense of awe and wonder at our own selves and our place in the whole.

What is beginning to emerge here, in Integral theory in general and in Integral Recovery specifically, is a vastly expanded field of understanding and depth that brings together the perennial wisdom of the past;[8] the wellsprings of the great spiritual traditions; and the scientific, modern, and postmodern understandings of cultural and individual evolution and development. As we noted earlier, our mental illnesses are characterized by rigidity and chaos, so we might also describe our cultural and historical illnesses as spiritual, philosophical, and economic rigidity and chaos. Again, the way to health, both as individuals and collectively, is through a process of integration. The emergent Integral health appearing in my students is shining a light and offering hope for our larger collective woes.

Being a guitar player, I can often tell if a young person picking up the instrument is going to be a guitar player or not. Those who have a passion for the playing itself are the ones who become guitarists. Many

For the Integral Recovery practitioner, every moment, every occasion, every incident becomes an opportunity to practice. With discipline, life itself becomes practice. The old joke about the tourist in New York who asks a local how to get to Carnegie Hall becomes our rallying cry: "How do you get to Carnegie Hall?" The New Yorker responds, "Practice! Practice!"

Before starting a practice session with students, I often ask the same question, "How do you get to Carnegie Hall?" The students yell back, "Practice!" Exactly.

will pick up the instrument for the promise of wealth, fame, recognition, or to be thought of as "cool." If that doesn't happen quickly, they move on to another field of endeavor, where the promises the guitar once offered may be fulfilled. True guitarists are the ones who fall in love with playing—the new discoveries, the familiarity, the valleys, the peaks, the plateaus, the fellowship of other guitarists. At fifty-five, I look back on my forty years of playing with warmth and gratitude that I stuck with playing long enough to reap the rewards of a lifetime of dedication to a form of artistic expression. I have recently realized that the quest for technical skill (both in my playing and in my singing) and competence has been transcended by the quest to bring forth soul, that deeper expression of my relationship to, and connection with, the world. (Although I still find joy in improving my technical skills on the guitar and writing new licks and songs!) Recently, I have been experiencing my guitar playing as yoga or even as prayer. Mark Williams, my friend and sometimes producer, told me that when he drums, he is sending the beats to God.

One of the keys to my personal success as an Integral practitioner has been very simple. The busier I am, and the more stress I am under, the more I practice. When life is easy and running smoothly, I can get by very well with my one hour a day of meditation and my five visits a week to the gym. However, when things get harder, I practice more. This works beautifully. Often, I have seen people fail and relapse because they say, "Oh, I'm too busy to practice." This is absolutely the wrong attitude and leads to failure. The harder it gets, the more I practice.

I was recently talking to a young man who was hanging onto his sobriety by his fingernails, due to the fact that his girlfriend had left him and was sleeping with one of his best friends. He was understandably very distraught and told me he had already meditated his hour in the morning. I told him to meditate for two more hours and call me back. He did, and he said, "Okay, I'm better." That's how it works.

I also want to be clear that one can be a part of our postmodern, fast-moving world and still be a daily Integral practitioner. The last few years have found me traveling extensively in connection with my Integral Recovery work, both in the United States and abroad. I have found that I can absolutely keep up both my physical exercise and my meditational practices while I am traveling. Airplanes are an excellent place to get in a good two- to three-hour BWE meditation session. Hotel rooms offer a great opportunity for continuing yoga practices, push-ups, crunches, and so on, and I am always on the lookout for gyms in whatever city

I find myself. On long road trips, I find that seeking out local gyms far surpasses loading myself up on caffeine to stay alert and feel good, and workouts make for nice, healthy breaks during a trip. I can attest that Europe has wonderful gyms available in every country I have traveled in. Jogging through new cities in new countries is a fascinating way of exploring the territory. I think of it as "touro-jogging." And, of course, I do my meditation first thing in the morning, no matter where I am, as I have my portable meditation temple in my iPod in the form of my Profound Meditation Program tracks. I have found that by keeping up my practices when I travel, I stay much healthier, and the grind of travel does not wear me down nearly as much as it would otherwise. I also find it satisfying to practice what I preach in keeping my practices going no matter the challenges of the circumstances.

Because the idea of lifelong practice is at the core of Integral Recovery, I want to examine some of the principles of practice and mastery as taught by George Leonard (1923–2010) in his book *Mastery*.[9] Leonard was an aikido master and teacher. In fact, he began practicing aikido in his sixties and achieved his fifth-degree black belt. He also co-authored, with Michael Murphy, the book *The Life We Are Given*,[10] which is the founding document of the whole idea of an Integral Transformative Practice, which Wilber and company later called Integral Life Practice—combining practices that work and engage the body, mind, heart, and soul simultaneously. It is an amazing book, and the authors deserve great credit for being some of the giants whose shoulders we stand on as we proceed into the world of Integral Recovery.

There are five keys to mastery that Leonard unpacks in his book, which we will cover here, examining their tremendous applicability to our task, namely, defeating addiction. Let's look at some of the things that we will need in order to gain mastery, or continued health, growth, and sobriety. Leonard's definition of a master is not someone who is really good at a particular skill or practice, but one who sticks with the practice. This is the heart of the matter, so we will look at some of these elements.

The first key is *instruction*. This means that one has to be willing to be taught; one has to be willing to learn from those who know more or who are farther along the path of mastery than we are. This requires humility and honesty. "I don't know what I am supposed to do, or how to stay sober; therefore, I am willing to listen to people who do." As an old AA friend of mine once told me, the attitude in early recovery needs to be, "I don't know anything about recovery. I'm the stupidest person in

the room, and I'm going to shut the hell up." Actually, the original version
of this wisdom was a bit spicier; my friend was from the streets of New
Jersey. There is, however, a lot of wisdom in this; a beginning student of
anything requires humility. One has to admit, "I don't know what I'm
doing." If one is not willing to be a beginner and look somewhat awk-
ward and silly at first, there will be no sobriety, no mastery. Just being
receptive to a teaching is a transcendent event. For example, a person in
recovery who emerges out of the drug-induced narcissism of egocentric
red now says, "All right, how do I do this?" instead of the usual, "Screw
you! Don't tell me what to do!" This is a major developmental leap in
attitude as well as altitude and should be acknowledged, supported, and
praised by the Integral Recovery treatment team.

Since Integral health care providers are on the path of mastery
themselves, they reach a degree of proficiency that allows them to teach
and speak from the authority of their own study and practice. This is a
key point in the Integral Recovery model: health care providers are dedicated IRP practitioners themselves. Because of this, I believe, there is an
actual transference of energy from teacher to student, which enlivens and
charges the student's weak batteries. Integral teachers also model just what
an IRP can produce. The reaction? "Wow! If that's sobriety, I want it."

Perhaps most important, an addict can sense if you're the real deal;
it's the old adage, "You can't bullshit a bullshitter." In my experience,
addicts are masters at detecting disingenuousness and can smell hypocrisy
in authority figures like bloodhounds. Building and establishing trust
is foundational in a successful treatment program. If the teacher is not
authentic and authoritative, the program will not work, and make no
mistake, the students will test the teacher. This is actually good and healthy,
but the teacher must stand ready to meet the challenge.

The second key to mastery as delineated by Leonard is *practice*. Or,
as the Sufis teach, the goal of spiritual practice is not altered states, but
altered traits. This is an essential understanding that we teach our students,
and the realization of this principle becomes a powerful initial motivator for disciplined practice. In the early stages of an Integral Recovery
Practice, it is natural that the practitioner is looking for results and relief
from suffering. But as recovery progresses and evolves, the practices and
the journey become the goal.

In my earlier writings, and in the first draft of this book, I often
referred to Tiger Woods as an example of dedicated practice and mastery.
According to almost all accounts, Tiger Woods' dedication to the sport

of golf was practically superhuman and way beyond what his contemporaries were doing. But now we know that this is not the whole story. So, while Tiger was a master of golf, he failed to practice and master other parts of his life. In fact, in one interview with him after his fall from grace, he said that he had stopped taking care of himself and that he had stopped meditating.

I believe we can draw many lessons from Tiger Woods' example. First of all, his dedication to practice over many years, instilled by his father, a former member of the Special Forces, allowed for Woods to become a golf and sports superstar. However, I think we can safely infer that Woods' practice was not an Integral practice. In other words, although he worked the body line, he may have not been working his mind, emotions, spirit, and of course, ethical line. This caused the collapse of his marriage, the tarnishing of his reputation, and the loss of hundreds of millions of dollars in the divorce settlement: ultimately, his almost supernatural skill at golf has not returned as of this writing. So whether we are masters of golf, the guitar, surgery, or any other skill, in order to maintain the healthy foundation of the skill, we must also embrace a practice that is Integral, that includes the five essential lines, body, mind, heart, soul, and ethics. In my case, I am absolutely sure that practice in these essential areas has allowed me to excel to a much greater degree in other areas of my life, such as music, writing, teaching, and relationships.

There is an interesting anecdote about Ben Hogan, the greatest golfer of his era.[11] When asked by a reporter why he was such a great golfer, Ben responded, "I'm very lucky." The reporter said, "But Ben, you practice more than anyone I have ever seen." Ben replied, "Yep, the more I practice, the luckier I get."

The third key to mastery is *surrender*. For the addict this means surrendering and accepting the fact that you do, indeed, have a disease and that without help and treatment, you will most probably die as a result. Also, unless the disease is arrested with help and treatment, it is only going to get worse. Surrender also entails surrendering to your teacher: doing what you are told with willingness, humility, and gratitude. In Eastern Orthodox contemplative work, this process is known as kenosis, which means emptying or letting go of all of our desires and agendas in order to be open to God, or our greater purpose—in this case recovery. We become willing to go to any lengths to accomplish this purpose, as the *Big Book* of AA teaches.

The last aspect of surrendering is to the practice itself: the ebbs and flows, the peaks and plateaus, the deaths and rebirths that are part and parcel of vertical-stage growth, as new stages of the unfolding Self emerge. Each time this happens, there may occur a sense of loss and grief as the old structures and concerns are left behind with no real certainty as to what the new territory is going to look like. This is surrendering to the process and the rapid evolution of stage development that a dedicated IRP is likely to produce. At times, hard-won competencies have to be given up in order to embrace the new skills required at the newly emergent level.

Eventually the feelings of loss induced by stage growth begin to subside, as one comes to accept and embrace changes that occur from a dedicated Integral practice. We can even welcome the death and rebirth of our old structures, because we realize that each developmental move up the ladder brings a new reorganization at a higher level of functioning. As Hegel said, all levels are adequate, but the higher levels are more adequate.[12] At the higher altitudes, we can see more, we have greater capacity, we can do more, and we have the ability to take more perspectives, which allows us to function in the world with more skillfulness and wisdom.

Difficulties that arise in conditions of rapid vertical-stage growth could be compared to the state in which a high school senior finds himself when he would prefer to remain a senior rather than start over as a freshman in college. Being at the top of the heap in high school can feel secure, "cool," and worth hanging onto. He might even consider flunking the grade and remaining a senior, but soon the "coolness" would transform into a pitiful state of being developmentally stuck. There's nothing very cool about being a thirty-year-old high school student.

This dynamic is very prevalent in recovery; the addict is, in many ways, in a state of arrested development. Over the years, I have noticed that if you begin the addictive process, say, at the age of fifteen, and get sober at thirty, you have often missed fifteen years of developmental growth; in many ways, you are emotionally still a fifteen year old and intellectually still an adolescent. For many of my students, just the reality of day-to-day living, holding down a job, going to school, paying bills, taxes, and so on, is a new and very challenging experience. In other words, some essential lines have a lot of catching up to do. Physically, you may be more like an unhealthy fifty year old. Unsurrendered addicts do not get well, just as unsurrendered practitioners do not achieve mastery.

A fourth key to mastery is *intentionality*. In Leonard's work, intentionality has to do with vision, character, and will power. In Integral Recovery, intentionality involves all of that as well as techniques for releasing outdated thought forms and replacing them with new, more optimal thoughts, beliefs, and visions of what we are and who we can become.

Earlier we said that one of the five causative factors that we have to address, in order for sobriety and recovery to endure, is our negative beliefs about ourselves and about reality. Kulkowsky and Peniston's work[13] offers amazing evidence of the power of visualizations and affirmations, coupled with low brainwave states, to reprogram and revolutionize the outcome of treatment. The basic underlying truth here seems to be that the brain doesn't recognize the difference between actually doing something and seeing or visualizing it in your mind. Visualizing something is one thing, but visualizing something in a deep meditative state seems to facilitate a fundamental shift in our felt and lived realities. Here, suffice it to say, if you want to manifest something, you must see it, taste it, and sense it in the mind's eye first; you must envision, or intend, the desired result. The master practitioner is a master of envisioning.

A recent personal experience might serve to illustrate the point. As my fifty-first birthday was approaching, I set my goal at being able to bench press 300 pounds. My birthday came, and I was able to do 285 pounds, but 300 was not happening. A little over a month later, after continuing my workouts, I was ready to try again, only this time, I visualized myself doing it the night before. I imagined the blood filling my arms and chest, strength energizing my lift, and saw the bar and the weights fly off my chest. Driving to the gym the next day, I held the same images in my mind's eye. Before I made my attempt, I breathed deeply and saw the same images. Finally, when I actually did the lift, the 315 pounds seemed to spring from my chest in a way that seemed almost supernatural. I had very little awareness of the weight, but I clearly felt a tremendous surge of focused energy.

Another personal experience might serve to illustrate the point in a slightly different manner. A number of years ago, I wanted to quit smoking. I was convinced that it was not a good idea for my health, wallet, or spiritual work. I decided to visit my parents, who are nonsmokers and can smell someone who has been smoking at 15 feet, to bolster my desire to quit smoking. I also told myself that each attack of craving was an attack by a corporate Darth Vader, who wanted to steal my money and my soul and eventually kill me in a slow and painful death. So, instead of getting overwhelmed, I'd get pissed off and could resist.

I found that each craving episode was simply a wave that would rise and dissipate, and the more time I put between myself and the last cigarette, the smaller and less powerful the waves became, while the time between each craving episode grew longer. I have taught this same technique to my students: change your stories and realize that each hour clean, each day clean, each week clean is a victory, and it gets easier.

The fifth key is called "*the edge*." The master practitioner is the one who has become her practice and has mastered the plateaus, the incremental gains, and even the setbacks. The edge comes when we bring absolute concentration, focus, and even zealotry to our practice. The great masters in sports are those who show up early at the gym to train, who give their all in every aspect of training and then stay late, do a few more laps, shoot a few more free throws, walk through a few more *katas*, and do a few more sets. And when the game and the lights are on, in whatever field of endeavor, and it is time to step up and rise to the occasion, the master is ready. The hundreds of hours of focus, concentration, and extraordinary effort come together, and the master acts with seeming effortless grace and skill. There is a great line in the Bob Dylan song "A Hard Rain Is Gonna Fall" in which the poet says, "I'll know my song well before I start singing." When you have traveled the path of mastery, when the time comes to give your gifts, you are *on*, and the game plays you. *There is no effortless grace of the master without the extraordinary, disciplined effort of the practitioner.*

Another key element of practice is pushing yourself to the zone of discomfort and even failure. This is the place where true growth can occur. For example, when practicing to master a musical instrument, you don't just simply pick it up and plink away and play a few notes or chords that you already know; you continually push yourself to learn more complex patterns, chords, and rhythms. And when learning a new song, or a new riff, although you are unable to do it for the first few practice sessions, with time, repetition, and deliberate, slow practice, you can almost feel the growth and restructuring going on in your brain, as the new abilities begin to emerge. It is, however, important to recognize this zone and not to push yourself beyond the failure zone to the panic zone. For example, if I were bench pressing 125 pounds, I would not move to 400 pounds for my next challenge, in order to stimulate my growth, strength, and ability. However, I certainly might work with 140 pounds. Over time, you will begin to sense your way (it will happen at a different time for each of us) as you become more skilled and more familiar with the ebbs and flows and nuances of ongoing, dedicated practice.

In addition to Leonard's five keys to mastery, there are four types of practitioners that he identifies. The first is *the Master* herself. This is the person who practices for practice's sake, as in, "That's what buddhas do!" The progress of the master is represented by plateaus punctuated by sudden upward blips; blips are followed by another plateau, slightly higher than the last one, but a little lower than the highest part of the last blip. When we love the plateaus and the daily practice, progress happens.

The next three types are the types that don't make it. Again, this is of mortal concern, because "not making it" in the case of recovery can mean relapse and death. So let us look at the approaches to practice that don't work. There is *the Dabbler*—a person who is infatuated with the newness and the rapid results one sees at the beginning of a practice. "Wow! This is great. I can't believe it." But then comes the first plateau, enthusiasm wanes, practice ceases, and, in our case, relapse begins.

In an Integral treatment program, clients are treated with kindness and respect and immediately begin a variety of therapies that help them feel better in short order. During the first week, we just want clients to begin to understand that sobriety feels better than the roller-coaster ride of addiction. The Dabbler will be delighted because progress comes very quickly at first. It is when the soon-to-follow plateaus kick in that the Dabbler loses his initial enthusiasm and ceases to practice.

Our highly technological society has become very addicted to quick fixes, whether they are technological, medical, or mood altering. In most cases, the quick fixes just don't work, especially on the deeper issues where our lives and humanity are concerned. The ability to Integrally practice over time builds persistence, willpower, hope, and character—all virtues and strengths that are pathologically missing in the person suffering from the disease of addiction.

The next type is *the Obsessive*. This is the bottom-line type, one who wants results and wants them now. Obsessives love breakthroughs and quantifiable results. They will push themselves hard and then freak out when they hit a plateau—not to mention a valley or a trough. The Obsessive does not understand the necessity of the plateau in development. This is problematic and very closely related to addictive behavior. "I want it, and I want to feel it now!" There is a story I heard once about the perfect drug. It was akin to a combination of cocaine, ecstasy, and heroin in its effects and lasted eight hours. It cost only two dollars a pill. The only problem was that it took eight hours to feel the effects! No addict would want it. "I want it now" is the attitude and the overpowering desire of the reptilian brain. That is the bait and the allure of drugs as well as alcohol—the song of the siren, if you will. You can feel good right now. You don't have to wait. The states that drugs and alcohol offer are quick and, in the short term, relatively cheap. Stages, however, take work: plateaus and blips, plateaus and blips.

Interestingly and encouragingly, practice is the opposite of addiction. In the beginning of the addictive process, the addictive substances or behaviors are extremely gratifying but lose their power to bring satisfaction and joy as the progression of the disease continues. In other words, it takes ever more of a drug to get the desired results, while the effects grow less and less. In the case of practice, however, the more accomplished one becomes, the greater the joy and satisfaction. The better writer one becomes, the more joy there is in writing. The better singer one becomes, the more power, depth, and enjoyment there is in singing. And, in the case of an art form, the recipients of the artist's gifts are also transformed by the level of skill that the artist has accrued through his or her years of dedicated practice. Think of the works of the great painters, musicians, writers, and sports figures whose skills have thrilled and inspired us over our lifetime. Then think what it must be like to be able to perform at that level. Extraordinary.

The third type who does not achieve mastery is *the Hacker*. The Hacker, after getting the hang of things, will be satisfied with the plateau. He paddles only enough to tread water. So, this type paddles for a bit, then quits and sinks. The Hacker is one who is satisfied with half effort and mediocrity. This type of practitioner, and hence his practice, is simply not transformational and will often be left behind. Transformation takes hard, concentrated, and sustained practice. It is through pushing ourselves beyond ourselves, on an ongoing basis, accepting the tremendous power to transform that each of us has and realizing a sense of responsibility for using that power for our greatest good, that radical and profound transformation occurs.

In a good treatment program, the initial phase can be dramatic, as the client moves from pathological addict-red back to the stage of development she had attained prior to the onset of the disease. Though the client now reinhabits her prior stage, there is still plenty of horizontal translation work to be done, such as dealing with the causative factors that led to the use and abuse of the drugs in the first place. Simply being back in the place she started from is obviously not sufficient, as that place was also the starting place of the addiction. So there is a lot of cleaning up and strengthening work to be done at the prior stage of development. As one Integral Recovery practitioner expressed to me, "I am currently doing the rather unexciting and unsexy emotional shadow work, such as vacuuming under the couch and cleaning under my bed." In other words, he was not engaged in spectacular and dramatic developmental growth, but doing the day-to-day emotional and shadow work to strengthen and beautify his current stage development. This is so important: falling in love with the mundane and undramatic parts of our daily practice and not becoming attached to the spectacular and the dramatic. In other words, we have to be comfortable with the highs, the lows, and the plateaus.

These three approaches to practice, the Dabbler, the Obsessive, and the Hacker, need to be recognized and skillfully dealt with in developing a client's IRP. We all probably embody each of them at certain times. For the addict, any of these attitudes toward practice can lead to failure, relapse, and death. I often ask my clients, "How much time did you dedicate to staying high?" The honest answer is usually, "All of it." So how much time does effective recovery take? The answer, in the initial phase, is again, "All of it." The work, therefore, of Integral Recovery in the initial stage, after detox and stabilization, is to establish a lifetime IRP as the axle upon which one's life turns. One's healing and sobriety depend on practice, and this will shape one's character and one's destiny.

In Shawn Phillips's Strength for Life model, he also charts a course from discipline to mastery, in which he lays out four stages of motivation.

- Stage One is obligation-based motivation, which is character-ized by "I should." This would be our Integral Recovery client that shows up at the door disheartened, despairing, and feeling like crap. He knows he needs to change, though he doesn't look forward to it, but he will allow us to help him through this initial stage.

- The second stage is called desire-based motivation, which is characterized by "I want to." This is the phase when the student looks around and sees the health and strength of his guides, teachers, and instructors, and says, "I do want this. I want to be healthy again, and I want to be stronger and feel better than I ever have." Here the motivation is strengthening because the goals are becoming clear and defined. These goals will grow and broaden as one climbs the developmental ladder of one's life.

- Stage Three is enjoyment-based motivation, characterized by "I love to do this." At this point, one looks forward to one's time in the gym, for example, simply for the challenge and the exhilaration of it.

- The fourth and last stage that Shawn calls Mastery is characterized by "I'm inspired—just try to stop me!"

So, what I am saying, and what cannot be emphasized strongly enough, is that extraordinary talent and greatness and exceptional recovery do not occur by dumb luck. They are the fruits of dedicated, deep, and deliberate ongoing practice. We must be able to answer the question, "Why do I practice?" And we must be able to answer the question, "How do I practice?" And, "What occurs when I practice?" For example, one of the greatest detriments that I have found to an ongoing meditation practice is what I call the meditation superego. This kicks in when you think you know what meditation should be, but when it doesn't happen the way you think it should, you become discouraged and quit. Obviously, we all want results, but the results that we are looking for will only occur with sustained effort over time. Live practice, do practice, be practice. Build friendships and communities and relationships with other practitioners that will support your practice and inspire you with continued growth. When I speak to my friends, clients, and former students on the phone or on Skype, my first question is always, "How's your practice?" That gets the ball rolling.

I believe that as more and more of us understand the absolutely essential role that practice plays in our own personal health and development, as well as our future as a species, we will enter into a whole new period of human history. I agree with cosmologist Brian Swimme[14] that we are in a place between stories. The old stories are not sufficient. They are like buckets with holes in them that just don't hold water anymore. New stories are emerging of survival, healing, and transformation, made possible and facilitated through extraordinary and dedicated Integral practice.

Let us listen to the voice of George Leonard, master teacher, aikido master, and pioneer of Integral Transformative Practice: "I believe that our failure to develop our potential is one of the most dangerous tendencies on the planet. Crime and war [and addiction] can be attributed to our failure to develop the potential of the vast majority of people. The main aim, shall we say, of all this work is to make it possible to develop your divine, God-given, universal potential. You've got no time to study war [or take drugs], if you are developing your potential. You'll be too busy to get into that kind of trouble."[15]

Religious scholar Houston Smith says, "Positive affirmative transformation is not just self-contained or self-centered. It improves the individual but it also improves all of the individual's relations, including the community as a whole."[16] The work we do on ourselves is work we do on the world. Just as a disease is a contagion and spreads, so does health and affirmative transformation. As I told one of my students early in his recovery process, "By the way, this is not just about you." To which he replied, "Oh, yeah, I forgot."

Service

We need to bring forth our gifts in response to life and in service to our times. If we don't, our "living water" will grow stagnant and unfit to drink: that which is within will poison us as it putrefies from lack of outward flow. If there is a healthy *self*-interest in service, this is it. As it says in the Prayer of St. Francis, "It is in giving that we receive."

There is an unofficial tradition in AA that recognizes that from the beginning of the recovery journey, a person must engage in service, even if it is in simple acts like showing up a few minutes early to set up chairs before a meeting or making the coffee (the nearest thing AA has to a sacrament)—simple, small acts of service that are an outward manifestation of an inward turning away from the egocentric black hole of addiction. As one's capacities grow, one is expected to increase one's degree of service by helping other alcoholics and taking part in the governance of the AA community at a local level and then at higher levels. This is one of the great insights of AA that is brought forward in the Integral Recovery model. As it says in Step Twelve of the Twelve Steps of Alcoholics Anonymous: "Having had a spiritual awakening as the result of these steps, we tried to carry this message to alcoholics, and to practice these principles in all our affairs."

In Integral Recovery, I express the idea this way: as a result of this awakening journey, I commit myself to a life of integrity and service. This, I believe, is covering the same ground, but it expands the circle of service and concern beyond other alcoholics, to include whatever one's particular callings are and whatever conditions are confronting one in life.

But let me add a cautionary note here: our service needs to be grounded in an ongoing Integral Recovery Practice. If it is not, our endurance and effectiveness will not be sustainable in the face of seemingly overwhelming needs and challenges.

In the late eighties and nineties, when I lived in the San Francisco Bay Area, I was very involved in social activism and saw many people around me fall under the weight of the load of this type of service (myself included) without an effective means of repair and renewal. The results of deeply committed service without a renewing practice are exhaustion, depression, giving up, and growing cynicism. Service should be the outward fruit of your inner work. Practice without service is eventually simple narcissism, and service without practice is self-defeating at best. At its worst, service without practice actually hurts the people and the cause you are attempting to serve. This has long been talked about in activist circles, but I believe that with the emergence of Integral practice and the Integral wave in general, a healthy and more balanced service ethos is now possible. In my mind, not to do my IRP is a selfish act, as I would decrease my effectiveness within and without. It is a simple moral imperative: *to live well, we must serve; to serve well, we must practice.*

As we empty ourselves with service and expressing our deepest gifts, we are renewed and refilled by our practice. This point is essential and cannot be avoided as one's life and practice unfold. In the beginnings of treatment and recovery, the capacity for service may seem small, but simply showing up is the first step. Service and practice are woven into the pattern of the Integrally recovered life from the very beginning of the recovery process in order for the foundation to be strong and the roots healthy. Alignment and integrity happen when our inward moral intentions match our outward behaviors. "We make a living by what we get, we make a life by what we give" (Sir Winston Churchill).[17]

13

The Family Component

Including families as a part of treatment is certainly not new, and the best programs that I have worked with have always included some version of family treatment. First, let me state the obvious: the disease of addiction does not occur in a vacuum, and the family is most definitely involved, sometimes as a causative factor and other times as a victim of the disease—sometimes both. In any case, to see one's loved one change from their former beloved personality to a manipulative, lying, hateful, Mr. Hyde addictive personality is incredibly painful for those who love the addict. There have been volumes written about "codependency," and many have said that the disease of addiction cannot continue and prosper in the absence of some sort of codependent and enabling support system. In other words, the family, by covering up the addictive behaviors and softening the consequences of the addictive, acting out behaviors (i.e., bailing the addict out of jail, making excuses for her tardiness at work or school, etc.), is simply postponing the day of reckoning. It often takes a great deal of work for family members to recognize these patterns and understand that they are not helping their loved one, but prolonging the suffering and supporting the progression of the disease. When we encounter a loving, distressed, but supportive family, we will definitely support and coach family and friends as they make the hard decisions to confront the addict with their behaviors and hold them responsible.

On the other end of the spectrum, there are families who are actually a fulcrum of toxicity and abuse. These families are not loving or caring, and their main problem is not enabling or codependency; rather there can be physical abuse, sexual abuse, emotional abuse, both the passive and active sort, or some combination thereof. There may be generational histories of alcohol and drug abuse and toxic relationships, and in such families, addiction is often the ocean that abuse swims in. At times, the "identified patient" (IP), or the one who is in treatment, can actually become the spark of health and recovery that can lead the whole family toward recovery. At other times, this is no longer possible; perhaps the family members are dead or at such a late stage of deterioration from the disease that they are unable to participate in any family or recovery work themselves. Most often, a family is somewhere in between these two points on the continuum from a generally healthy, supportive family to a completely addicted, abusive, pathological family.

Family conditions must be accounted for and dealt with. We can help our student accept her past and deal with the conditioning and trauma that her family of origin has created in her life, or we can hopefully enlist the entire family in its own healing process. When doing so, the Integral provider must function as a coach, offering hope and inspiration to begin the healing work and practices. These practices include a myriad of different interventions according to the needs of the individuals in the family group. Bottom line: it is great to have the whole family adopt an Integral Recovery Practice lifestyle. In addition, individual family members may need individual therapy, couples counseling, and ongoing family therapy. Often Al-Anon meetings can be of great help. These are 12-step-based meetings, where an addict's family members and loved ones go to deal with their own wounds and the pain associated with being in intimate relationship with an addict or alcoholic. One of the most useful things about such support groups is that, in this context, a family will have the dawning recognition, oh my God, we are not alone; millions of other families have gone through this same experience. Also invaluable is that here families can learn the difference between supportive love, which holds the addict accountable and responsible for his behaviors and his recovery, and codependent, or enabling love, which allows the disease to continue its progression and continue to cause suffering in the lives of the addict and those in relationship with him.

Please note, there are meetings, and there are meetings. In other words, some meetings are vibrant, inspiring, and supportive, while others . . . not so much. Just as when you are looking for a church or spiritual community, for example, you must do a bit of shopping until you find one that is appropriate for your current spiritual needs, likewise, you may need to look around before you find the Al-Anon or Alateen (Alateen is for younger family members), or any 12-step meeting for that matter, that is a good fit for you. So, don't base your opinions on one meeting. You may encounter an excellent meeting right away, but sometimes you will need to look further.

More often than not, addicts will be dragged kicking and screaming into treatment. This early attitude, interestingly enough, does not seem to have much effect on the eventual outcome of treatment. Remember again, we are dealing with at least two personalities here: the addict self, who really just wants to take drugs, and a more genuine self, who wants to get well, but who is in an extremely weakened state and not the dominant force in the ego at this point in early recovery. Thereafter, with love, tears, practice, and hard work, the motivation changes from "I have to do this" to "I want to do this"; the addict has become self-motivated. This is a great turning point in treatment.

In treatment, as in raising children, both mother love and father love are necessary. Mother love holds a suffering addict in absolute acceptance and compassion in the light of what we know about the disease of addiction. This means accepting you for who and what you are and understanding that although you have done bad things, you are not essentially bad. It is the disease of addiction that causes people to act out in ways that are truly harmful. The hurtful acting out and other criminal behaviors are symptoms rather than causes. Mother love holds the addict in the compassion of this understanding.

Father love, on the other hand, deals with these symptomatic behaviors and holds an addict accountable for his actions and responsible for taking charge of the recovery process. Father love will not support you if you choose to leave treatment or continue a lifestyle that ensures continued access and use of drugs. Father love will not support you financially while you continue to use. Father love will write you out of his will, if necessary. Father love might change the locks on the door. Father love requires guts, courage, wisdom, and a very deep love indeed. It is this father love, more often than not, that gets the addict to the dance of recovery. By the way, father and mother love are not gender specific but can be administered by either gender or even by the same person. The art of knowing which type of love is needed when and in what measure is something that takes wisdom and experience to learn. Hopefully, IR practitioners will be in a position to provide this skill and understanding to the families they work with.

One form of tough father love is when law enforcement, the justice system, and treatment facilities work together to induce an addict into treatment. Law enforcement and the justice system can hold the addict responsible for her criminal behavior and, at the same time, provide the necessary motivation to get the addict into treatment. In other words, hard work (in treatment) or hard time, your choice. Once, I was asked

how I get newly recovering addicts to do brainwave entrainment meditation, and I somewhat jokingly responded, "Meditation or jail, what's it
going to be?" This is often not far from the truth and is an example of
ruthless father love.

Mother love loves you no matter what; father love loves you when
you do the right thing. Children need both to become healthy adults.
They must internalize a healthy self-regard and the acceptance of the
mother and at the same time have a sense of healthy shame when they
misbehave and do not live up to their highest potentials and core values.
In IR treatment, both of these types of love must be present; again, the
art is in learning to balance them as needed and appropriate.

For an Integral health care provider, both types of love need to be
included in one person, so we don't play good cop/bad cop with addicts.
In early recovery, mother love is more important; just as in the early life
of a child, mother love is more important than father love. Clients must
feel that they are accepted, welcomed, and cared for. But as treatment goes
on, and health is restored, the balance between mother love and father
love begins to shift, and our clients become responsible for their own
healing process and held accountable to the high standards it requires. If
there is just mother love, the whole process becomes weak and narcissistic.
If there is just father love, the process can become too authoritarian, and
clients' behaviors can become inauthentic, in other words, just focused
on looking good in order to gain approval.

When I co-founded the wilderness program Passages to Recovery,
I made it very clear that when a new student arrives in the group, he is
to be welcomed with camaraderie, love, and a great deal of acceptance.
This was borrowed from the wisdom of AA, which states that the most
important person in the group is the newcomer. Prior to that, in other
wilderness programs I have worked with, newcomers were often isolated
from the group in the first days and only allowed to watch and listen to
the other group members, while being fed a rather simple diet, different
from what the other group members were eating. While I understand
the philosophy behind this approach, I feel that such isolation is contraindicated in the case of addicts and will only reinforce the shame, loneliness, and fear they are already experiencing. More often than not, being
dumped in the middle of nowhere with a group of people you've never
met before is hard enough. This is an example of mother love being used
initially to establish relationship, connection, and trust before the boot of
father love is strategically applied. Over and over in my experience of

treatment, I have seen that trust and compassion must first be established as the ground from which the rest of the work will grow and emerge.

In working with families who are often located in different parts of the planet, a trusting relationship can be established on the phone, or preferably online, using Skype or iChat, where you can actually see the person you are communicating with. I personally have found this to be a *great* leap forward in the treatment field, as the difference between looking at someone while conversing is tremendously more connective and intimate than merely talking to a disembodied voice on the phone. In fact, I have developed very close bonds with people I have never been in the same room with using these methods.

For an IR provider, establishing a relationship of trust and caring often consists of asking questions, listening to the answers, and showing sympathy and empathy to the suffering family. This empathic and sympathetic listening can be enhanced with reflective listening techniques such as, "I can feel how deeply you love your son and how painful this has been for you all." Once a relationship of empathy and trust has been established, one can begin moving the family toward beginning their own healing process. Most often, this starts with them establishing their own Integral Recovery Practice. When coaching IRP online, I first establish what the needs of the individuals are, physically, emotionally, and spiritually. Then I start the family members on their own BWE-enhanced meditation practice (20 minutes every morning, for the first two weeks, followed by 40 minutes every morning thereafter). This is a very good place to start, as the individuals usually begin to feel the transformative power of BWE meditation quite quickly and become more willing to do the other practices, such as adopting new nutritional and exercise regimes. This also creates a firm and supportive foundation for the family member who is in treatment, as in, "You are not alone in this. Your family is doing this too." This is the kind of commitment and cohealing work that gets results. The families that practice together, evolve together.

Teaching family members to develop their own Integral Recovery Practice is an essential and perhaps revolutionary part of Integral Recovery. As the first noble truth of Buddhism teaches, life is suffering. Anyone born in a human body has issues and suffers, whether it is addiction or something else. In my early days of forming Integral Recovery, when I shared the IR model and practice with an old Christian gentleman, who was also an M.D., he paused, looked at me intensely, and said, "This is not just for addicts, is it?" Indeed, it is not. I once had a parent tell me that whether her son chose to get better or not, she was going to get better due to the practices that she had learned. In Integral Recovery, families learn new ways of dealing with and supporting their addicted family members, new ways of working on themselves and improving their own Integral health, and new ways of communicating that allow for open and honest communication.

Following is an outline of the progression of events that typically take place between Integral Recovery treatment providers and the family members of an addict who comes to IR for residential treatment.

We begin working with the families from day one, as most often it is the family that contacts us first about getting help for their family member. One of the first things we have the family members do, if they haven't done this already, is to download Skype, so that we can use it as our primary communication channel. As stated earlier, I believe that Skype and similar technologies are really changing the way we live, communicate, and do business. This is certainly true in the business of Integral Recovery.

So from the beginning we establish a close working relationship with the family. We get a history of the addicted family member from the family's perspective, and we ascertain what their financial situation is (sufficient funds makes all of this much easier). Historically, insurance companies have not liked to pay for treatment. In fact, they seem not to like to pay for anything. So, coming up with the monies necessary for treatment is often very challenging.

The next step usually involves doing an online Skype interview with the perspective client or Integral Recovery student. If the student seems appropriate, and everything necessary for the student to enter IR residential treatment falls into place, we're on. During the student's stay with us, there is an ongoing educational process with the family. First of all, we ask them to watch Dr. Kevin McCauley's DVD *Pleasure Unwoven*. This explains, very eloquently and in an easily understood manner, that addiction is a brain disease. This is often a revelation to the family members as well as the students. We also have the family members read *Integral Recovery*, so they begin to understand the practice and the basics of the AQAL map that we use with our students. Then we have family members begin to use the Profound Meditation Program, as this is very useful in helping them to deal with their own stress and wounding. It also creates a sense of "We're all in this together, and we're all working on ourselves." We let the family members know that treatment, getting well, and staying sober is a lifelong journey. And we tell them that the work we are doing in the first phase of treatment is establishing a healthy foundation for the student, giving her the tools and understanding that she needs to stay sober and to continue growing in a healthy way.

We recommend that family members attend some local 12-step meetings and Al-Anon meetings so that they can begin to understand the disease of addiction from the mouths of other addicts and alcoholics. There they can also learn about their part in the family dynamics and how to play a healthy role, rather than the role of enabler, or outright rejecting the student because of her past addictive behaviors.

During treatment, our therapist, in this case my wife Pam, makes weekly calls to family members to continue educating, working with, and appropriately supporting them. After the first month, we usually shift to weekly family therapy sessions via Skype, with the therapist, the student, and his family. Then, in the last few days of primary residential treatment, we hold what we call the Family Workshop.

The Family Workshop

At this point, the family and the student have been apart for the duration of primary treatment, and now it's time to bring them back together again to continue the healing process. What follows is offered as an inspiration and as a guideline, but not as an immutable given; in other words, this family workshop component will continue to grow and evolve as does the Integral Recovery model in general.

The first morning, when the family members arrive, we invite them to participate in our morning routine, which consists of yoga and meditation. This is probably the first time that the family members have meditated together; it is often very powerful and reinforces the understanding that practice is something for everyone. After meditation and breakfast, we usually spend the rest of the morning with the families but without the student, so we can answer questions about aftercare and review the AQAL map and the disease model of addiction in person. I am a firm believer that repetition is the law of memory and that going over the basics again and again is very helpful and very reinforcing.

In the afternoon, in what is perhaps the highpoint of the family workshop, we do what we call the 4 Rs. This is something that we have instructed both the student and those family members who will be there for the workshop to prepare ahead of time and bring with them to the workshop. The 4 Rs are Resentments, Regrets, Respects, and Requests.

- Resentments are the things that they resent that the other person (in this case the student) has done to hurt their relationship. For example, "I resent that you stole so much of our money to buy drugs." And the student might say something like, "I resent, Dad, that you were never around when I was growing up."

- Regrets. This portion is a time for each individual to acknowledge regrets for the things that he or she has done to hurt the relationship. For example, the student might say, "Dad, I regret that I stole your money to buy drugs." The father might say, "Son, I regret that I wasn't around more when you were growing up."

- Respects. This portion is where everyone acknowledges the things they respect about each other. For example, the student might say, "Dad, I respect how hard you worked to support our family." And the father might say, "Son, I respect the hard work that you have done in this program to heal and get sober."

- Requests. The last part is simply things that each individual requests for the ongoing relationship. Note that we say request and not demand.

This is the setup. We have the family member and the student sit in the center of the room facing each other with just a few inches separating their knees, and it is very important that they maintain eye contact while communicating the 4 Rs. We normally start with the student, who begins with his first R, "Dad, I resent that you were . . ." We have the father maintain eye contact and reflect what he just heard. For example, "Son, I hear you resent that I was not around while you were growing up." This is not a time to defend oneself or to make excuses, but to simply practice reflective listening. It is not a practice in winning an argument or convincing the other, but in clearing the air and teaching healthy communication skills. As this is going on, Pam and I are present, acting as facilitators and coaches during the process.

It is also important that each one of the Rs be short and concise as it takes away from the impact and becomes hard to follow if they are long rambling paragraphs instead of short and brief sentences. During the resentment portion especially, it is helpful if each individual uses specific examples. For instance, "I resent that you stole my grandmother's silver to support your drug habit." Using specific examples makes the process more powerful. After each round, we have the other family members who are also present, as well as the Integral Recovery staff, offer their reflections and feedback. For example, "I was really moved when you said . . ."

As simple as this process is, it is very profound. Most often, there has been a lot of hurt and many things that have never been spoken or acknowledged. Much healing can take place when we can deeply listen to one another without justifications or incriminations. After this process, the family spends the rest of the afternoon and the evening together and begins the work again the next morning.

The next morning we begin again with our yoga and meditation practice, and we go over the aftercare plan, relapse prevention, triggers and warning signs, and what happens if relapse does occur. Whenever possible, we recommend that the student go from our treatment facility to a long-term sober living environment, which is a less structured living environment in an urban setting, where the student can go back to school, or find a job, while at the same time live in an environment where she is held accountable and there is continued support for staying sober.

One of the most dangerous times for students is immediately after leaving primary treatment. They have been practicing hard and living in a very supportive and safe environment. It can often be a shock on the system to go back to the world, especially if it involves the old grounds and playmates of their using careers. This produces great stress on the system and can be a powerful relapse trigger.

When it is not possible to send the student to a secondary treatment center, we try to build in a strong support system. This often includes getting an AA sponsor, attending meetings, and continuing counseling sessions with me or Pam via Skype twice weekly. It is essential that students incorporate their Integral Recovery practice into their lives as, again, relapse begins when one stops practicing.

It is very important that the first year of recovery be very intense and focused and that sobriety is put in first place. As Bill W. said in the *Big Book* of AA, "Half measures avail us nothing." Just as addiction, in its latter stages, is a full-time job, so is recovery a full-time job, in the early years. It does get easier with time, as one builds new habits and new ways of living.

In our second-day morning session, first the IR student reads his Relapse Prevention Plan, which might include 12-step meetings, continuing meditation practice, and other details such as carrying a list of

phone numbers of people whom the student can contact if he is beginning to think about using. (By the way, we also have our students go
through their cell phones and delete all their using friends and dealers.)
Other Lower-Left quadrant support elements of a Relapse Prevention
Plan will include the groups and organizations that the student will join
or participate in to support his healthy, Integral Recovery lifestyle, such
as churches, temples, mosques, meditation groups, and Integral Practice
groups. The Relapse Prevention Plan may also include continued therapy
with Pam or a local therapist and ongoing family therapy.

Next, the student reads aloud his list of triggers. These are events
or objects that may provoke a craving response in our students and raise
the risk of relapse. This could be certain neighborhoods, such as where
the student used to score drugs, liquor stores, certain people, certain
music, and certain objects or paraphernalia, such as pipes, baggies, spoons,
lighters, hypodermic needles. A trigger can be something as simple as
the clinking of ice cubes in a glass. This list of triggers helps reinforce
wise choices for the student and also gives nonaddict family members a
deeper understanding of what it means to be an addict.

We then review warning signs, which the student has also listed.
These are signs that perhaps relapse has happened or is getting ready to
happen, and action steps must be taken. Common warning signs are "If
I begin to isolate again; if I begin to be angry and manipulative; if I
start lying; if I stop practicing; if I stop going to meetings," and so on.

Last but not least, if relapse does occur, generally the first thing
is to get back into primary treatment. If it is just a slip rather than a
full-fledged relapse, then other less drastic responses might suffice. But,
most often, when relapse does occur, it is not subtle. One of the very
mysterious things about this disease, as I have mentioned earlier, is that
though there may have been a substantial period of sobriety, it seems
that for the addict the disease has continued to progress, even though
he has not been using. And when an addict does begin using again, he
wants to make up for lost using time in the first few days. This puts the
individual at great risk of overdosing.

Families and Developmental Stages

One of the huge, if not revolutionary, contributions of Integral Recovery is adding the vertical developmental line to the recovery map. This

knowledge is *essential* for working with families, as we will often have families at different developmental levels, for example, a traditional values/ blue family, a family with primarily modernistic orange values, or a counterculture green family. To make the situation even more complicated, you might also find that various family members are at different levels, such as a blue mother, an orange father, and a green son. Talk about a lot of fun and variety! At this point, one must begin to develop the skill that Integral teacher Jeff Salzman calls simulcasting. This means that after a short period of time in conversation with said family members, you can discern what developmental level each family member is speaking from. If you simply speak to the needs and the concerns of one family member at his level, you will tend to isolate the other family members very quickly. So you must learn to switch back and forth, gracefully, to speak to the concerns and levels of each member. If you are really good, this can seem effortless, and even be effortless, but it takes a while to realize this degree of mastery. You could practice on your own family at Thanksgiving or Christmas dinner, or any other family gathering. This not only gives you first-person experience, but it also can be a test of your spiritual maturity when you feel tempted to strangle Uncle Bob. As Wilber has often quipped, if you think you are enlightened, go home for the holidays.

Eventually, as all family members, including the addict, begin to comprehend the different developmental levels, this understanding will also foster compassion, such as in, "Oh, Mom is so blue. That's just the way she is, and I need to respect and honor that." Or, "Oh my God, my son is a green hippie. I guess I'll just have to learn to live with and love that too." You can feel the drift. This knowledge can also lead to more humor and objectification of these different developmental attitudes within the family. We begin to be a little more compassionate, understanding, and accepting of our own and others' foibles and sacred cows (in the case of green, a sacred vegetarian cow).

Families and Enneagram Types

The Enneagram is an extremely useful and transformative lens with which to view not only ourselves but also our family members. It gives us a whole new understanding of our family dynamics. As Integral Recovery's main Enneagram teacher, Leslie Hershberger, says, we must not only pay attention to our own Enneagram points, but we are deeply affected by our parents' Enneagram points as well.

For example, I am an Enneagram type Six, my father is a type One, and my mother a type Three. As I began my inner journey in graduate school, I was rather shocked when I got to the part of myself that told me I could never be good enough nor could I ever do enough. As you might imagine, this made me feel very badly about myself. I was largely unconscious as to why I had such a poor self-image. Later, I realized that I had integrated my father's type One agenda, of being the perfectionist judge, so that I felt I could never be good enough, and my mother's type Three agenda, of being the achiever, so I felt I could never accomplish enough. Note that I feel I had very good parents; they were not consciously laying these burdens on me, but, in a very interesting way, I had picked up on their inner scripts and made them a part of mine. As I became aware of this and worked through these levels of my conditioning, I became freer and happier with myself. At the same time, I was able to retain the healthy ethical part of my father and a lot of my mother's work ethic. I now see these parts of my inner inheritance as gifts and not as problems. This is an example of how understanding our families' Enneagram types can help us with our own inner work, not to mention better understanding our family members and being more skillful and hence compassionate in our relationship with them.

It can be particularly poignant for a parent to realize and accept the differentness of her son or daughter, through the Enneagram lens. A type Nine father, for instance, can have a type Eight daughter and recognize that it requires a different style of interacting in the relationship, than if his daughter was also a Nine. An Eight, because of her power focus, needs to feel met energetically, and a more passive Nine can actually raise anxiety in an Eight, which then leads the Eight to become aggressive, which can consequently lead to all kinds of challenging family dynamics. So a type Nine father learns that he must call up the strong, powerful part of himself to interact successfully with his daughter and release the Nine tendency to avoid or withdraw from his intense daughter. This is one example, but it illustrates how useful the Enneagram can be in helping us understand how to be more fully present and engaged with people, when we know their particular personality dynamics and how those interact with our own.

14

Relapse Begins When You Stop Practicing

Addiction is a chronic disease that often involves relapse. Our ultimate goal in Integral Recovery is to change this, but, for the moment, this is what we have to deal with. So what can we do to prevent relapse from happening? In Integral Recovery and in relapse prevention, the AQAL map is the key, and Integral Recovery Practice is the hand that turns the key. To stay strong, healthy, and sober, we must make sure that we are taking care of business in all the essential parts of our lives. If there is dysfunction in any of the four quadrants, steps must be taken, when possible, to correct those issues. If we are experiencing problems in any of the five essential lines, we must take steps to rectify those deficits and adjust our practices so that all five lines remain at a high and extremely functional level.

We must also make sure that we are taking care of our housecleaning at our current stage of development and that we are expressing our current stage in the most positive, wise, and compassionate manner that we are capable of. And we must be aware when stress and neglect of our practices and our own essential health lead us to stage regression, where we behave in an unhealthy manner at a moral stage that is lower than one that we have already achieved.

We must be sensitive to our emotional health, dealing with our shadow and emotional wounds from the past, as well as dealing with the new issues that we are tempted to push into the shadow and the hurts that are a part of the day-to-day experience of being alive. Again, our ongoing Integral practice will make us ever more skillful in achieving emotional health.

Finally, we must be aware of our personality typologies in order to maximize our strengths and minimize the negative effects of those areas we are challenged in. An ongoing and deepening understanding of typologies, specifically the Enneagram, will give us the knowledge and skillful means to be much more effective in all of our relationships.

Clearly there will always be problems and issues that, even through our best efforts, we will not be able to change or make better. An approach to this is well-addressed in the portion of the "Serenity Prayer" used in AA work, "Lord, grant me the serenity to accept the things I cannot change, the courage to change the things I can, and the wisdom to know the difference." We can, and should, make positive changes in all four quadrants as we go, but there are some things outside of ourselves we will not be able to change, which can be sources of tremendous stress. What do we do about them? The simple answer is that we accept things the way they are. Given this, do we just sit idly by and accept? By no means! We practice.

We must understand that the key to our health, evolution, greatness, and sobriety is in our own hands. While at first this may seem daunting, we eventually get beyond that to the empowered and inspirational realization that, yes, we can become and be more than we ever thought possible. Through our Integral Recovery Practices, we can transform ourselves from being another tragic statistic and victim of the disease of addiction to an exemplar of a fully actualized and realized human being, at the forefront of leading our human family through the shifts, changes, and growth that we so desperately need to navigate these difficult and challenging historical times.

How do we prevent relapse? By becoming master practitioners. Besides our own personal practice, here are two key issues that must be considered and incorporated into an integrally recovered life:

1   It's not just about you. When our health returns, and our capacities begin to grow and come online, we must make ourselves available to serve our fellows. Whether this is working with other addicts or any other myriad of suffering beings is up to the individual and his own conscience and inner sense of direction. But we must work on this service ethic and practice kindness and respect in all our dealings with others. If we don't, we will miss a great opportunity to see the beauty and sacredness of each individual, no matter what her current stage of development, and our soul will become crusty and clogged with our own narcissism, which in itself can be an important factor leading us to relapse and the downward spiral of the disease of addiction. To put it simply, egoism, selfishness, and self-centeredness are contrary to the

spiritual attitude and health that we need to permeate our lives in order to maintain our sobriety and continued growth.

2. We must pay attention to our Lower-Left support system. In other words, we must cultivate healthy relationships with individuals and groups that will support our goals of Integral health, sobriety, and service. The negative side of that coin is that we cannot, in the language of Alcoholics Anonymous, continue to hang out with the same old playmates and in the same old playgrounds that supported our drug use and addictions. In other words, don't go looking for your local support group at the local pub or drug den.

Community is essential. This can be a healthy religious organization of your choice, 12-step meetings and support groups, Integral practice groups (that you may have to start where you live), or simply having workout partners who will inspire you and support you in your physical practices. It is also important to make sure that your romantic relationships and liaisons are with people who are like-minded and supportive; I have often seen people's sobriety crash on the rocks of unhealthy romantic relationships. And we must seek out professional help whenever necessary in the areas in which we need support, which could include individual therapy, family therapy, nutritional counseling, personal trainers, pastoral counseling, and so on. It is very important, when seeking the help of a nutritionist or therapist to make sure they are savvy when it comes to alcoholism and addiction.

But again, I return to the most basic truism of Integral Recovery: relapse begins when you stop practicing. In addition to that, something I have found to be true in my own life and in the lives of my students is that in times of increased stress, one must not only not neglect one's practices, but *increase* the amount of time and attention paid to one's practices.

For example, a few family visits ago, things were not going well when I was at a family reunion. We were rubbing up against each other, and it was becoming difficult to keep things on an even keel in a loving and kind manner. During this visit, I increased my meditation time to an hour and a half a day and got up before anyone else was awake to go exercise. While this did not alleviate the difficulty, it did facilitate the experience to become one from which I learned a great deal about myself and my early childhood conditioning. The dots started to connect, and I began to understand some of my habitual ways of acting in the world, which had often played out for me as a resistance to authority. (I am the youngest child.) So I stayed open, felt the pain, and kept observing what was going on in my relationships and what was going on inside of me. Shortly after this rough visit, I called the family members with whom I had the most problems and apologized for my behaviors. I assured them that I was not looking for an apology from them but was truly apologizing for what I had done; and I affirmed how much I loved them.

This practice, which was carried on in subsequent family visits and has evolved and improved over time, seems to have shifted my family dynamic. I feel that my relationship with my family is now much better than it has ever been. We love one another and enjoy one another and have become much more expressive in our love and appreciation of each other. This is one example of a stress situation in which dedicated and even increased practice can serve as a catalyst for improving the whole gestalt, or web of relationships.

As an interesting note to this experience, I heard one teacher say that when we are doing our individual practices, we can actually hold the pain of a whole system, in this case my family, in our hearts as we practice.[1] This is a powerful meditational technique that will certainly increase our compassion and understanding as we do it. It is akin to the Buddhist practice of *tonglen*, where one breathes in the pain of the world and breathes out loving kindness. Whether this, in actuality, helps heal others, or simply transforms the individual doing the practice, is not clear; however, I am certain that when we work on ourselves and become wiser and more compassionate, and we act from this place, we can often shift the gestalt or dynamic of the whole group.

Every pain, every hurt, every relationship is an opportunity to practice. To be totally present and open, allowing the situations and hurts to deepen us, is really a radical way of looking at life's challenges. As a friend of mine said, "Don't say, 'Oh shit!'; say, 'Oh, fertilizer.'"

Here follows an example of how relapse occurs when we stop practicing. This was fresh in my mind when I completed the first draft of this book, and, during that time, an inner voice that sometimes speaks to me quite clearly during my morning meditation said, "Write your tears." So, here are my tears and thoughts on relapse and its prevention.

I had just returned from a wedding of a friend and former student. The wedding was an elegant and grand affair in a setting that made me think of *The Great Gatsby*, 21st-century style. There was a lavish amount of food and drink in an incredible, newly built mansion on the water's edge. It was a black tie affair that made me wonder what the heck I was doing there. I soon found out.

My friend, whom I shall call Abner, was getting married a few months after completing treatment—too soon, as he was still in early recovery. The ceremony began in a room that looked like a modern Gothic cathedral. Things were flowing nicely, and I had never seen Abner looking so handsome, healthy, or radiant. Then I noticed that as part of the ceremony there was going to be communion served: bread and wine. At first, this didn't register. And then it did. When I saw what was developing, I broke out in a cold sweat. Part of me felt that I was watching a Greek tragedy play out. I knew the end of this story. I wanted to scream out, "Abner, stop! You can't drink!" But I didn't. Another part of me was saying, "It's just one sip. It is, after all, sacramental . . . Maybe God will give him a pass on this one." I should have shouted from the balcony, "Stop!" to save my friend's life. But I held my tongue, and I failed my friend.

Exhausted by the whole experience, I returned to my room, took off my rented tuxedo, changed into clothes that were more comfortable, and then rejoined the festivities. By the time I returned, the best man was making a speech about the groom, and Abner was toasting him with champagne. Spirits were high, the evening still young and full of laughter and promise, and Abner was in full relapse and in mortal danger.

Relapse does not begin with the first drink or the first ingestion of the addictive substance. Like addiction itself, it starts out as a small thing: a thought. I was a binge drinker . . . one little sip couldn't hurt . . . it is, after all, sacramental. Didn't Jesus say to remember him in this way? And so forth. Where did the relapse start with Abner? Where does it start with anyone? It begins when one starts taking short cuts with one's IRP. I'm too busy today. First, I have to work myself out of this financial hole and then I'll have time to practice. I've changed; I'm different now. It's my freaking wedding! It's sacramental! It's the most important day of my life! I've been so good, I deserve it. Don't be such a fanatic! One drink can't hurt . . .

I left the party early that night. The next morning when I saw Abner I could smell the booze on him from five feet away. I told him that I needed to talk with him, and we went off alone. The rationalizations and denial began. The relapse was total. I then began my 10-hour drive back home. My heart hurt. Addiction − 1 : John − 0, I thought. As I have said before, I take this very personally. Addiction (and alcoholism) is a relentless, wily, and at times baffling opponent. To win against such an adversary, one must be skillful, strong, and understand the adversary well.

In Abner's case, we arranged for him to go right back into treatment, which he did. He then returned to his wife and family, renewed and humbled, and has been an amazing success story ever since. Fortunately, Abner married a very wise and strong woman, who was eager to learn about the disease that was afflicting her new husband and was fiercely supportive of his program of sobriety.

Again, to be successful, Integral Recovery must be grounded in a lifelong Integral Recovery Practice. Why? Because addiction is a chronic brain disease that involves relapse; therefore, treatment and practice must last a lifetime. The first 90 days should be at a residential recovery facility (sorry, 28 days are not enough; this arbitrary number was set by insurance companies that didn't want to pay for more). Here one establishes one's IRP, to include work on all the causative issues enumerated earlier, and starts to clean up one's messes and work toward a healthy balance in all four quadrants. For the next nine months, the first year being crucial to long-term recovery, our recovering individual should live in a healthy, sober environment that supports an Integral practice-based lifestyle.

Not everyone will be able to live in a designated secondary treatment center or halfway house, as often people must return to their families, jobs, and so forth. But whatever the best available living situation, all the necessary supports need to be built in. In other words, someone just out of primary care can't live with a roommate who is using drugs or alcohol, or smoking cigarettes, for that matter; it just won't work. Even if the other person is not an addict, it is too much for a newly recovering person to be exposed to these triggers. Clients will need counsel on how to achieve a supportive living situation from Integral Recovery support staff and should use an IR guide or coach, which could also include a more traditional 12-step sponsor, on an ongoing basis. As I have often said elsewhere, addiction is a powerful and ruthless disease, and we cannot deal with it in a haphazard or half-hearted way and expect to get the results that we seek. Again, dedication, wisdom, and humility, which means the willingness to seek out and take the advice of others who know more about long-term sobriety than we do, are essential qualities that must be used and cultivated.

During the secondary treatment period, for the alcoholic there should be daily Breathalyzer tests, and for the drug addict professionally administered drug tests every three days (no home tests, please; the possibility of false positives is substantial). Just as the diabetic must check her blood sugar and insulin levels daily, so does the addict's continued sobriety need to be confirmed. If relapse occurs, and on occasion it will, the client needs to return to primary treatment until the treatment team agrees he is ready to return to a less structured environment. All of these safeguards must be agreed upon and established before the client leaves primary treatment. This is to avoid hemming and hawing, manipulation, and drama. Relapse occurs; the plan kicks in; the client returns to a higher level of treatment. This level of intensity and verifiability needs to be in place for the first year of sobriety.

After the first solid year has been achieved, the danger of relapse occurring decreases to a great extent. This doesn't mean that relapse doesn't happen for those who have even many years of sobriety. I have often heard tragic accounts of people who have been in recovery for many years, including trusted leaders in AA groups or other 12-step programs, who have relapsed and in many cases died. What seems to have occurred in these cases is that there were serious shadow issues that had not been dealt with and that their re-emergence was too much for the individual to handle. Hence, their relapse and death. It is my growing belief, based on experience, that the shadow practice and emotional work that are a core part of the Integral Recovery program will lessen, if not eliminate, these tragic occurrences.

I have been studying the phenomena of relapse for years, and while it is painful to watch, it is predictable and needs to be handled objectively and compassionately as part of the recovery process, in most cases. Traditionally in AA, it has been said that it usually takes three or four relapses for stable, lasting sobriety to be achieved. Obviously, this puts the addict at risk, and sometimes these relapses can prove fatal, as often happens with heroin addicts who go through treatment and then go out and use again. When they inject the same amount of heroin that they were using before, they overdose and die, not realizing that their tolerance has lowered while they were in treatment. This is a common occurrence among heroin addicts and should be talked about and explained during treatment.

But often, relapses are temporary steps backward and do not negate progress made prior to the relapse. Sobriety is cumulative, and the work adds up, even when there are temporary regressions. AA supplies many pithy and powerful bits of wisdom, and one of my favorites is, "It's hard to have a belly full of whiskey and a head full of AA." In other words, once you have achieved a degree of Integral health, some of the sheen and romantic luster is taken from the siren's song about drugs, and a return to drugs is seen for the dead end that it is.

What I said above about sobriety being cumulative is also true of Integral practice in general. Even if we fall off and stop doing our practices, when we pick them up again, we are not starting from square one. The work we have done before is still with us. And though our bodies and brains may be a little out of shape, they will get back into shape and function at a higher level more quickly than if we had never practiced at all. The time and effort spent in deep Integral practice is never time wasted.

Let me be clear that, in most cases, when an individual is in the latter stages of the progression of the disease of addiction, and the compulsion to use and take drugs has become the overwhelming purpose of the individual's existence, extended residential treatment is very much desired and usually required. However, I have been able to do some very successful work with individuals who are at a stage where they feel they are beginning to lose control over their consumption of alcohol and drugs. They may still have most of their life intact—such as marriage, jobs, and parenthood—but they are beginning to experience a fear of losing that which they care about most. In these cases, each one of which must be considered individually, I have found that individual counseling and coaching can work very well. Because of the advent of the internet, and wonderful technologies such as Skype, I am able to do this work with students from all over the world. I also make it clear at the onset that if this coaching relationship, in which the student is supported in developing his or her own Integral Recovery program, does not work, then we must reevaluate and consider if a residential treatment program is required. This usually becomes clear within the first few weeks of working together.

In the initial coaching session, I listen to the individual's history and concerns and give him his homework assignments, which usually start with reading this book and beginning to use the Profound Meditation Program. He starts out using the first track for 20 minutes a day, gradually increasing this over time, and from there implementing the other Integral Recovery Practices. I have found that BWE meditation leads to very powerful therapeutic inroads into students' issues and processes, usually quite early in the process. At times, for example, students suspect that there are issues or events in the past that led to their drug or alcohol use and abuse, and, at other times, students are very clear about what happened in their past but have not been able to do the work necessary to release and heal their traumas. Here, a combination of the Profound Meditation Program, coaching on how to do the release work, and more supportive traditional talk therapy might be indicated. In either case, I have found that the BWE meditation works as a powerful catalyst for this healing to happen and as a powerful lubricant to the gears of explorative talk therapy.

In a very practical sense, when thoughts of using begin to re-emerge—when our life stressors are waking up the reptile, and the barbarians are at the gate, while the gate is giving way—what do we do? I have prepared what I call the Integral Recovery Relapse Prevention Tool Kit, to train my students what to do when these situations arise—and they will.[2]

The Integral Recovery Relapse Prevention Tool Kit

1. Double or triple your meditation time. Switch into Witness mode and allow whatever feelings arise to fully present themselves in the light of mindful awareness. Let them have their full expression and release them. As a part of this process, 3-2-1 shadow work may be very helpful.

2. Keep allowing the feelings to be present until they pass. In fact, welcome them as the raw fuel for your continued growth and liberation from suffering.

3. Get to the gym or hit the trail running with all the intensity and discipline that you have developed from your ongoing Integral Recovery Practice. You will almost always find relief and feel better.

4. Do a cranial electrical stimulation session for the next few days to support optimal neurochemical balance.

5. Do not isolate. Hang with those who know what is going on and will support your efforts to deal with the stress and upset in your life. This also includes having a list of phone numbers of people whom you can call for support with your sobriety. In the twenty-first century, we are all very connected and available to one another; let's use this ability in a good way.

6. Know that every time you meet a challenge and win, you are that much stronger and fit to triumph in whatever life has for you.

7. Have a list of sober friends in your wallet, your purse, or on your cell phone, whom you can call for support when you find yourself in a dangerous situation or when you are beginning to feel cravings to use drugs or alcohol. It is important that you have a number of these sobriety friends so that if you cannot reach one you will be able to reach someone else. Also, just the act of calling someone for support is a step in the right direction and can actually help break you out of the addictive trance.

So there it is. You can also customize and add other tools to this kit as your journey evolves, and you gain more experience in dealing with these situations. Please share what is working for you with all of us who are involved in Integral Recovery and are on the cutting edge at this time. You have a plan and powerful new tools that no other generation of recovering people has ever had at their disposal. Use them wisely, courageously, and with gratitude.

With the advent of iPods, smartphones, and similar devices, we can carry our meditation practice with us wherever we go. I have found that travel has become a great opportunity for more practice and not less. For example, one can almost always take a meditation break and sit for 20 minutes until an episode has passed. The cravings and temptations are not a defeat but an opportunity to practice and triumph. Again, remember that practice is cumulative, and even small periods, where one sits down and goes inside, can have a powerful healing, centering, and transformative effect.

I also recommend that, under the threat of relapse, you practice BWE meditation for three hours for the first couple of days. This will show you that you can indeed meditate for longer periods of time, and you will also experience the power of longer meditations and the push that one gets from such heroic effort. You will actually feel your meditation getting qualitatively deeper and deeper; a lot of stuff gets released and worked through.

Another tool of great importance is the understanding that relapse is a process. Relapse does not begin with the ingestion of the substance. First, there are seductive thoughts about taking drugs; in the recovery field, this is called "euphoric recall," and it feeds the addict's desires and cravings. In euphoric recall, one only remembers the good things about using: the warmth and the burn of the first shot of whiskey, the rush of relief when the heroin hits the brain, or the blast of pseudodopamine when the line of cocaine is snorted. During these recollections, one forgets the awakening in abject physical misery, the depression, the betrayals, the lies, the broken relationships, the utter loss of control, and the accompanying despair and depression.

This is when 12-step meetings can be so helpful, because when one hears another's story, one recalls one's own history and remembers that everything the addictive substances once promised were just mirages, leading not to paradise but to a wasteland. However, one does need to be very much on guard against what is known as "war stories" in treatment, because there is a very fine line between telling one's drug history and beginning to glorify the high. Drug talk can trigger a chemical reaction in the brain of the newly recovered; then cravings begin to take over. Thankfully, with time and healthy recovery, the individual becomes less vulnerable, but it is a very real danger to the newly sober.

At Passages to Recovery, we used to say, "Behavior is recovery—sobriety is behavior," when we saw a behavioral relapse occur, even in the absence of substances. (Just as morality ultimately comes down to what you do and not what you think about doing.) An attitudinal relapse, characterized by familiar addictive behaviors such as anger, lying, manipulation, and self-centeredness (the angry, egocentric red personality), if unchecked, eventually and often quickly leads to chemical relapse. The best antidotes to this behavioral and attitudinal slide down the spiral are the healthy virtues of gratitude, humility, and acceptance, along with a renewed dedication to one's Integral practices and living as though one's life mattered.

So relapse does not begin with use, but with the thoughts about using, brought on by specific triggers, with remembering the good things and self-censoring the bad, and, of course, lapsing in one's practices as one begins to entertain the seeds of these thoughts. It is important to note that an addiction is not just to the substance itself, but also to the rituals and objects associated with using. Standard procedure in treatment identifies the different triggers that change one's brain chemistry, in order to stop the chain reaction from trigger to thoughts to cravings to using. In IR treatment, students are instructed to write out their own warning signs, which will signal, both to themselves and to others, that either relapse has occurred or the chain of events leading to using has begun. This is why treatment providers say that if a student is going to maintain his sobriety, he cannot go to the same playgrounds and hang with the same playmates that he had during his using career; the triggers are much too powerful. Triggers actually change the brain chemistry—just as one's mouth waters when seeing or smelling delicious food. These triggers can be extremely dangerous in early recovery, especially as they can initiate the whole sequence of compulsive acting out that leads to using again and relapse.

An Integral Recovery practitioner will know what to do when these triggers occur. The first thing is to limit exposure to the triggers—old using friends, certain music, liquor stores, certain films, books, almost ad infinitum. Each one of us has our own personal triggers. The first thing to do is leave the scene of the crime. If you are at a party, for example, and the cravings are kicking in, vacate the premises. Don't let false pride keep you around. The rule is sobriety first, and the rest will follow. If there is an event you have to go to where alcohol will be served, bring a sober friend with you as a support person. It is also recommended that you have a sponsor and several other sobriety support people that you can call on when in need. You could go to an AA type meeting, work out, meditate, do releasing work. It is essential to have sober friends, a community that is involved in spiritual growth, and Integral Recovery Practice.

Your Community of Healing and Evolutionary Growth: How to Put Together an Integral Support System

At the beginning of this book, I spoke about how the disease of addiction is a progressive, chronic, and, if not treated, terminal brain disease. As we have also seen, it is more than an Upper-Right brain disease; it is a disease that infects all other quadrants as well. This means that when a student finishes the initial Integral Recovery transformative treatment process, it is not the end of treatment. It is certainly the beginning of a new life, but the journey for an Integral practitioner never ends. Given this, each IR treatment center graduate needs, as a part of this very process, to build a support system and community that will facilitate his continuing practice and growth for a lifetime.

One of the advantages of the IR treatment program is that we have Integral Recovery coaching built in, which will support our students when they leave the container of the IR treatment center. The first month of treatment consists of showing up, beginning to feel better, learning the basic ropes of IR, and establishing one's practice. The second month involves deepening one's knowledge and practice. The third month involves beginning to teach some of what one has learned to the newer students, as well as deepening one's own practices and preparing for the transition to a new life away from the IR treatment center.

During the last month, students make contact with their IR coaches and establish a relationship that will be part of their support system when they leave primary treatment. It is highly recommended that a student return to the IR treatment center at least three times in her first year—to ground, reconnect, and inspire. One of the biggest mistakes that people often make when leaving treatment is having a sense of their own invulnerability, as in, "Now that I've changed, I can handle it." While I think that IR treatment graduates will be much stronger than most people coming out of primary treatment, there is simply no good reason to put oneself at this kind of risk, ignoring the need for ongoing coaching and support. As I have said before, old playmates and old playgrounds put one at risk. It is essential to find new playmates and new playgrounds that will support one's health and continued sobriety. As students go forward, things must be, and are going to be, different.

At this stage of growth in the IR model, our first generations of students, who will become some of our best and most influential teachers and guides, will be the original leaders of IR support groups and communities. Initially, we intend to offer every kind of support we can to help establish these communities and support groups wherever they are needed (which is almost everywhere). The primary focus of IR support groups is to support practice. Secondarily, they are a social group. But practice is the goal and the grail. Being Integral, our IR practice groups are actually appropriate for almost anyone who wants to do the work, whether they are addicts or not. As I have said previously, I am not an addict, but my deep clinical depression almost killed me, as it did my brother. I recently said to my meditation group, "You guys might think I'm very disciplined the way I've stuck with my practices, but I don't think I was that disciplined. I think I was that desperate." Like an addict, I could not have continued in my disease and survived.

The initial process of leaving the safe fortress of the Integral treatment center will be to establish the patterns of practice in your new life. This is one of the areas where your IR coach will be of great assistance. Just as a good football coach will motivate, correct, and even kick your butt if necessary, so IR coaches will be there for you. In addition to utilizing your IR coach through telephone or internet coaching sessions, or in person if possible, you will need to reach out to people and organizations that will support your Integral lifestyle. This could mean churches, synagogues, mosques, zendos, gyms or health clubs, yoga studios, and the like. Since there are not many Integral organizations out there, you will need to find different organizations for specific needs. One of the universal truths that one finds in all the great spiritual traditions or religions is the importance of a spiritual community and spiritual friends. We need others of like mind and like aspirations to support us in our Integral lives. We need one another. Most of us, with perhaps some very,

very rare exceptions, simply cannot do it alone. This means joining or finding communities and friends who will be there for us, who will support us, and who, in turn, can be supported by us. The other side of this coin is, again, you cannot hang out with people or organizations that pull you down. It simply will not work.

As with all of our Integral practices, finding and forming supportive communities takes work. Examples of professional individuals that can be sought out and used are therapists, both individual and family, meditation teachers, personal trainers, massage therapists, yoga teachers, reiki practitioners, and nutritionists. You can also find teachers and mentors to help you develop those particular lines that are not included in our Integral Recovery Practice but are part of your passion, joy, and life goals, such as music teachers, writing teachers, or whatever else your callings might entail. Remember, as Viktor Frankl said, if you can discover what you want to live for, you can always discover the how.

It is generally thought that the mastery of any skill, whether it is playing the piano, learning a new language, or becoming a master Integral Recovery practitioner, takes about five years. So do not get discouraged if, in your first month of guitar lessons, you are not rivaling Eric Clapton. It takes a while! But that is part of the joy and the glory. And know that anything worth doing is worth working for—with discipline and dedication. What I am saying is that there is no easy way out. But there is a way out; the way out is through, and it rocks!

Another truth I would teach to recovering students in therapeutic wilderness programs was that every time they helped the group, or did their part, or cooked a meal, or walked the trail with us, they were being of service to others. And that little outward flow of goodness they were giving us through their sincere efforts was part of their healing process. So, never forget, as your capacities grow in wisdom and skill, you will be called on by life, or the universe, or God, by whatever name, to be present and serve. Ultimately, our soul's satisfaction is not found in what we receive but in what we give.

So get ready to re-think, re-feel, and re-organize your entire life. This is a lot, I know. But your future will be very bright indeed, and the alternative is, well . . . very dark. One of the exciting things about being part of something new is that you are one of the founders. I have often thought that early Christianity was a hell of a lot more exciting than that which came 400 or 500 years later. So know that if you are called to choose Integral Recovery for your life at this time, you will be a pioneer and a forerunner of an unfolding that has a potential we cannot even imagine. Someone once said that it is easy to know how many seeds are in an apple, but we can never know how many apples are in a seed.

Again, all the great religions and spiritual traditions have recognized the need for community to support the spiritual aspirant. There is a powerful and very helpful field of energy generated by people who work and share and practice together. In Buddhism, the three pillars are (and every tradition has a similar version of this) the Buddha, or the Self; the Dharma, which is the teaching and the practices; and the Sangha, or the community of aspirants. Integral Recovery is the same: without the map, the community, and the practices, recovery simply will not stick. Without these three solid pillars in place, the roof will sooner or later come crashing down.

In closing this chapter, I would like to quote from Rumi, the great Persian poet and mystic.

> Come, come, whoever you are.
> Wanderer, worshipper, lover of leaving—it doesn't matter,
> Ours is not a caravan of despair.
> Come, even if you have broken your vow a hundred times,
> Come, come again, come.

I want Rumi to remind us not of the drudgery of recovery, but of the joy of discovery. Though we fall to our knees, regress, and relapse a hundred times, we pick ourselves up and continue, because we have seen, through our practice and the journey to our deepest selves, the radiant light of pure Consciousness. Our diseases, failings, sins, and foibles are all thinly on the surface of our true Self. In that Self, we are perfect and whole. Resting in that knowledge, we pick ourselves up, dust ourselves off, and continue the mysterious journey of the unfolding of our lives.

Afterword

I think the members of my generation, the baby-boomers, have a lot to answer for. In the late sixties, I saw drugs begin to insinuate themselves into my upper-middle-class junior high and high school at a time when the American Dream was beginning to seem empty and hypocritical. Many of my generation embraced drugs as a way to wake up, have fun, and thumb our noses at the older generation. We smoked our pot and shouted, "Hell no, we won't go!" as the older generation drank their alcohol and worried about the domino effect in Southeast Asia. We boomers saw the world anew in a glorious blaze of radical rock and roll, pot smoke, LSD, and anything else we could get our hands on to alter our consciousness. In a wild mix of idealism, drugs, some tremendous talent, and often fatal narcissism, we opened the Pandora's box of drug use and abuse, and the promise became largely a curse. We opened the door, and our children and their children have paid the price.

Perhaps with my work in developing Integral Recovery, I am attempting to pay off that karmic debt accrued by my generation, with our radical embrace of mind-altering substances, one life at a time. Perhaps the postmodern green wave, upon which my generation rode to adulthood, didn't have the necessary moral certitude and discriminating wisdom to confront the messes we had made. Perhaps our moral ambiguity gave rise to the highly politicized, right-wing, fundamentalist religious movement that has become so vocal and influential in our country in the last 40 years—the excesses of green gave rise to the excesses of blue. Our "anything goes" attitude did a lot to bring the formerly disenfranchised into the mainstream of American life, which is a good thing, but it is no way to raise children.

I live in a largely Mormon community in an area as isolated as one can get in the lower forty-eight, and, yes, we have alcohol and drug problems, but seemingly not so much as the rest of the country. *U.S. News and World Reports* reported our local high school as one of the best high schools in the country for getting its graduates into universities. Someone quipped, "It shows how desperate these kids are to get out of Wayne County." But I think it is much more than that. These young people are raised in a largely drug and alcohol free environment. Wayne County High School also excels in sports, often winning state championships in wrestling and baseball (not enough students for football). Some of this is due to the tough Mormon pioneer stock that moved into our valley in the mid-1800s, but I think it is mostly due to the fact that they are largely clean and sober.

I recall a biopic about Bill Wilson, co-founder of AA. In one of the last scenes, he is with the other AA cofounder, Dr. Bob, who is dying. They are both looking back on all that had happened and all they had accomplished founding and guiding AA in the early years, and Dr. Bob says, "All we had to do was stop drinking."

All we have to do is stop using. Time and time again, I have seen miracles of transformation happen, as I have helped to get people away from the contagion of drugs and into a healthy living space that allows them to heal and pushes them to grow. My hope is that, as the second-tier unfoldment occurs, growing out of the fertile soil of that which came before, we can transcend and include the discipline of healthy blue, the science of healthy orange, the compassion of healthy green, and, yes, the strength and ruthlessness of warrior red. Ken Wilber once said that a society has the right, nay, the moral obligation to protect its young people from life-destroying drugs. My hope is that in the coming years, as the Integral/second-tier level fully emerges as a player on the national and international scene, we can find a way that unites us in our diversity with the love, ingenuity, and strength that is inherent and available in the human developmental spiral. Perhaps, we can find that which unites us no matter where we currently live on the developmental ladder: the love of our children.

As we clean ourselves up and take back our world from this plague of abuse and addiction, we will include all quadrants, all lines, all levels, all states, and all types. Perhaps, in the future, our children will not have to say "no." In the meantime, we can begin with ourselves, and with courage, compassion, and masterful intrepidness, practice and make ourselves fit and capable to face the challenges of our times and lives, living not from shallow, narcissistic surfaces but from the enlightened depths of our human hearts, where the Holy Grail of wisdom and compassion that can and must heal our world abides.

My prayer is that this book, and the work that I and others are doing in this emerging field of Integral Recovery, will be a candle lit in the darkness of despair and that it will begin to roll back that darkness and create pathways of hope and healing for our people, whole nations, and the generations to come.

I love you all.

The end.

Appendix 1

On Becoming an
Integral Treatment Provider

As Ken Wilber has pointed out in his writings and talks on Integral Medicine,[1] it is not only the body and mind of the patient that matters, but also the consciousness of the physician. The consciousness of the treatment provider is particularly important in the addiction recovery process, since one of the first steps in treatment is eliciting the client's buy-in to the very notion of practice as a path of recovery. If the treatment provider is transmitting health and wholeness by his mere presence, it goes a long way toward attracting the client to own her own recovery process. "If this is what health and sobriety look like—I want it!"

Exhausted, burned-out healers are worse than none; they are actually impediments to a client's healing. Just as in the Marine Corps, where everyone's first calling is as a rifleman, whether one is a general or a private, a cook or a clerk, in an Integral Recovery program everyone is first and foremost an Integral practitioner. Not only does this keep the program healthy, inspiring, and flowing, but it also overcomes the dichotomy of "I'm an addict and you're not." The emphasis becomes growth and optimal health. "How's your practice? This is what I'm learning . . ."

It is important to remember that if the choice is perceived as a choice between depression, chronically feeling bad, and addiction, in almost all cases addiction will win. It is essential, from the very beginning, that the client see and sense that she is onto something that is much better than addiction. She needs to sense the health, happiness, and integrity of the treatment providers, in their depth of understanding, their caring, and their support.

Integral Recovery treatment providers adopt Integral practices not only to communicate a healthy presence to those in need of our help, but also because as we practice ourselves, as well as becoming physically, emotionally, and spiritually healthier, we become more creative, more empathic, and greatly more capable of opening our hearts to our clients and their suffering. As we, as Integral treatment providers, continue to work on ourselves, we also become more integrated in our own lives and less susceptible to the exhaustion and burnout that often accompany this type of work.

The extraordinary benefit of increased creativity and problem-solving ability, which comes from our ongoing practice and our daily BWE meditation practice in particular, allows us to see deeply into each individual situation and be able to flow with and respond to each individual's needs within the context of the Integral model. This is something that cannot be achieved merely by knowing the model; it requires showing up and doing the work. While there are great similarities in the overall recovery process (which is why AA meetings are so powerful for alcoholics because one hears one's own stories over and over again through the words and lives of others), each individual is different and has his own unique set of problems, challenges, and capacities. So our enhanced creativity and the ability to respond effectively to each new student, and as new situations arise, are great benefits of our ongoing Integral practice.

Another great effect of our practice is increased empathy, along with its healthy correlate, compassion. In working with those who suffer from addiction, and their families, there is always a great deal of suffering going on. If we do not know how to be present with this suffering, those whom we serve will sense this, and there will be an essential disconnect, which will affect trust and the healthy deepening of the therapeutic relationship among all concerned. Also, if we are open to this suffering but do not know how to deal with it in a skillful way, we ourselves will become overwhelmed. But through our inner work and our practice, we become ever more capable of being present with whatever arises, whether it is grief, anger, depression, or even great joy.

We learn to be absolutely open to all that arises, moment to moment, to simply be aware of and allow, not grasp or hold onto, our feelings. Our increased capacity for mindfulness and nonclutching empathy is an extraordinary tool that enables us to be very present and allows our students to know that they are not alone. Remember, the root of the word "compassion" comes from the Latin "to suffer with." As our abilities grow, emerging from our Integral practice, we "suffer with" our clients yet remain centered and healthy ourselves, and even increase our spiritual and emotional health, as our ability to be present and healthily compassionate deepens with time and practice.

Remember, too, when we practice and work on ourselves, it is not just our kinesthetic or body awareness, or our intellectual capacity, and it is not just our emotional intelligence, our spiritual depth, or our ethical clarity, but it is all these things together, the sum of all these healthy parts, that makes an extraordinarily healthy and brilliantly capable whole. We are qualified to take our students there because we have done, and are doing, the work ourselves—day to day, week to week, month to month, year to year. This takes us beyond the dichotomy of doctor/patient, therapist/client, sober/not sober, this/that, to create a new, more coherent and unified field of treatment, which allows for a much healthier environment and greatly increases the potential benefits of treatment for those we serve.

Jesus warned the religious leaders of his time that they should not place heavy burdens on their followers—ones which they themselves were not willing to take up. In the same spirit, we cannot, with integrity, ask of others that which we are unwilling to do ourselves. It simply won't work in the long term, and when we are out of integrity, it is very difficult to ask it of others. In the beginning this might seem a bit overwhelming and overly challenging, but with a little work and time, when we realize our own responsibility and ability to transform ourselves into ongoing, improved versions of ourselves, the journey and the practice become less and less of a burden and more and more an open-ended delight of self-exploration, creativity, and transformation.

Now that we have talked about the importance of our Integral practice, let's spend a little time talking about what it means to get Integral. The first step toward becoming Integral is to learn AQAL, or the Integral map. As I explain to my students when teaching about lines, it is most often the cognitive line that leads the way for the others. So just learning the Integral way of looking at things—seeing the four quadrants in every situation that arises; understanding multiple intelligences and lines and how they develop semi-independently (e.g., you can be extremely intelligent cognitively and an absolute disaster physically); learning stages of development (which can *completely* change the way you look at the world); learning the states of consciousness beginning with the basics, waking, dreaming, and dreamless sleep; and studying and learning about masculine and feminine types and the Enneagram—can change your life. As Ken Wilber says, "The AQAL map itself is psychoactive." I would further add that each part of the map (quadrants, levels, lines, states, and types) is psychoactive and transformative in its own right. When integrated, they can be life and world changing.

The following are good resources to set you on your way to becoming Integrally informed. First of all, there are Ken Wilber's books. *The Integral Vision*[2] is a very condensed version, and many have told me it is very helpful. See also, *Integral Psychology*.[3] If you want to go for the brass ring, learn the secret handshake, and win the secret decoder ring, go for *Sex, Ecology, Spirituality*.[4] For the less ambitious, the Integral Life website, integrallife.com, and integralnaked.org are excellent resources, full of articles, papers, video clips, and MP3 audio files. They provide a huge archive of some of the most brilliant teachers on the planet discussing the many aspects of the Integral vision. Have fun!

AA meetings can be important training tools, as well as NA meetings and MA meetings. I have listened to literally thousands of addicts' stories, and they have always been a source of wisdom and amazement. Just when you think you've heard it all, there's a new level of betrayal, and often depravity, that the latter stages of the disease of addiction can cause. One also learns hope—that millions of people can and do get well. As a treatment professional who is not personally an addict, I fill my talks and classes with statements like, "A former student of mine told me . . ." or, "I have heard other alcoholics tell me . . ." This informs the addict that you do listen and have been listening, and that you actually know what you are talking about. You can also use stories from your own life and the lives of family and loved ones who have been addicts. This emphasizes the point that, addicts or not, we have all suffered from this disease and all have a stake in its defeat.

Read, look, listen, and practice. In my opinion, to be an effective Integral Recovery provider, you must yourself be a master practitioner. You simply cannot effectively lead where you have not been willing to go yourself. If you are interested specifically in becoming certified as an Integral Recovery counselor or health care provider, we are developing a program to provide Integral Recovery certification. In the beginning, I think you will find that just starting to look at the four quadrants of each of your clients will make a huge difference in creating a more comprehensive and truly holistic approach to treatment and counseling. Are their bodies healthy? How are their interiors? How are their relationships? And, how are their survival, financial, and other Lower-Right quadrant issues being addressed? This alone, I feel, could cause a revolution in health care.

In addition to using the four quadrants, making a basic lines assessment of clients' core strengths and weaknesses, in other words their intellectual, emotional, spiritual, physical, ethical, and relational skills, is very important. If there are other lines issues, such as challenges making or dealing with money, these need to be considered as well. Also, assessing your client's developmental center of gravity is hugely important. If you are speaking green speak to an orange or blue client, you're going to have real problems establishing a beneficial therapeutic relationship. Remember, Integral Recovery is not just for people at an Integral level; it is what allows us to be more effective with our clients at any stage of development—meeting them where they are and where they live.

Incorporating states of consciousness is also essential, especially since we are using new brainwave entrainment technologies that deal with different brainwave frequencies, which correlate directly to different states of consciousness. We are living in a golden age of brain research and are discovering that the brain is inherently changeable, transformable, and evolutionary at its core. The more we understand this most essential and human of our organs, the brain, the more this will translate into a quantum leap in the quality of the healthcare that we are able to provide.

I believe addiction can simply and usefully be understood in terms of states: addiction is a compulsive drive to achieve certain states of consciousness and an absolute avoidance of other states. With this knowledge, we can better understand our clients' struggles, and by educating them that states are just states, neither to be avoided nor sought after, we begin building the foundations for a drug-free and emotionally healthy life.

Learning the basic typologies of masculine and feminine and studying such typological systems as the Enneagram and Myers-Briggs is another essential element in Integral treatment. For a masculine-identified client, many of his emotional and relational pathologies will evolve masculine, narcissistic, "I gotta do what I gotta do, and to hell with the rest of you" issues. With your more feminine clients, pathologies will typically involve giving themselves away unhealthily in relationships. Healing for the masculine, therefore, involves becoming more caring and relational, and for the feminine, it often involves achieving more autonomy.

Gaining an understanding of types is a tremendous tool for each individual's self-growth and understanding, as well as an invaluable aid in learning how to skillfully engage with others in the essential relationships in our lives. A deeper appreciation of types also helps us understand our own often unconscious ways of dealing with others—and specifically with

our clients. When we don't understand different types, we may fall into
the error of thinking what works for us will work for everyone. Different types have different essential core issues that must be dealt with in
different ways. A knowledge of types is a great aid in getting away from
an unskillful, cookie-cutter approach to treatment.

I especially recommend the Enneagram to increase our capacities
and skillfulness as Integral treatment providers, and there are many good
books on the subject (see references).[5] Dr. William Glasser[6] once stated
that there are a handful of relationships in our lifetime that are essential
for our happiness. How we deal with those relationships is one of the
most important things that we can work on to increase our own happiness
and effectiveness as human beings. I am convinced that the Enneagram
provides an extraordinary tool for achieving just that.

To summarize, and I hope that this has already become quite clear:
to be an Integral Recovery treatment provider, you must begin your own
Integral transformative process and journey. This is not just about "them."
This is about you and me and we. As science has taught us, and as the
great spiritual traditions have also clearly illuminated at the highest levels
of their teachings, we are all in the deepest sense truly one. At a very
down-to-earth, mundane, and practical level, we are deeply connected. I
might add that to heal you is to heal me. And to heal us is to heal the
world. One of my favorite principles and core values, which is perhaps
the core value of Integral Recovery, is that nobody is saved until we all
are saved. So get busy, and let's join together in transforming and healing
ourselves and, in doing so, facilitate the healing and deep transformation
of those who are in our care.

I would recommend getting started immediately on a daily brainwave entraining meditation program. For an early work on this subject
and other related technology, see the somewhat dated but still valuable
work of Michael Hutchison in *Mega Brain Power*. Also, see the website
profoundmeditationprogram.com, as there you will find ever more, continually updated content on the scientific basis of brainwave entrainment
technology, as well as how to skillfully use it. I believe you will find
this one step of beginning a daily BWE-enhanced meditation practice
to be extremely useful and satisfying. I have found that there is possibly
nothing more hopeful and helpful than the knowledge that we, through
our own efforts, can improve, heal, and better ourselves in a way that is
very effective, rapid, and absolutely discernible by the one engaged in
the practice. This is a core strength of the Integral Recovery approach:

that we can take responsibility for own healing and achieve extraordinary and sustainable improvements in our lives, our bodies, our consciousness, and our relationship to others in the world.

I would also recommend getting Shawn Phillips' book *Strength for Life*, Integral Institute's *Integral Life Practice Starter Kit,* and, for your spiritual work, studying Ken Wilber's CD collection *The 1-2-3 of God.* I have also found that *The Sedona Method*, by Hale Dwoskin, is an excellent resource as far as emotional releasing and spiritual work go.

Remember, all the practices and the wherefores and how tos that I have included in this book are not just for addicts. They are for all of us. They are especially important if you plan to be a teacher and a guide in this field. Don't delay. Get started today. One day at a time, and one step at a time.

Also, feel free to contact us at integralrecovery.com should you have any further questions in these regards.

Appendix 2

Integral Recovery and the Greater Field of Addiction Treatment

In my work, the question has arisen, "Where do I locate Integral Recovery in the greater field of addiction treatment?" As I mentioned in the introduction, this book is by no means intended to be the authoritative last word on Integral Recovery; rather we anticipate that the model will evolve and improve as we learn more about the many aspects of this disease. What Integral Recovery *is* intended to do is allow us to put the best that is currently available into the service of addicts and their families. The Integral map allows us to have a large and expansive overview of this disease and how it affects the individual, society, and the culture at large. It is expected that this revealing overview will improve the individual parts of this whole, just as the individual parts and practices will change our view of the whole as we develop them and deepen our understanding of each facet of the model.

There are two main aspects of this book. One offers very specific techniques and technologies and hard-won knowledge and wisdom about the treatment of addiction. The other, and perhaps equally important, aspect presents a model or a framework that allows us to include what we deem are the best of the myriad practices and approaches with which we can effectively address the problem in a truly holistic manner.[1] Why is this so essential? Historically, in this country, the problem of addiction has been left largely to 12-step-based support groups and law enforcement. While this approach has achieved some things, obviously it has not been enough since the problem of addiction continues to grow worldwide, and the war on drugs that began in the Nixon administration has proved a dismal failure in protecting our people, especially our young people, from the devastating effects of this disease.

Over and over again, I have queried doctors both young and old, as well as students currently enrolled in medical school, asking them what they are learning about addiction. The answers have been shockingly vacuous of any real content. I have heard answers such as, "Addicts are real problems, and we don't like to deal with them." Or, "Nothing." Or, "Well, there certainly are a lot of medical students who are using amphetamines to study . . ." I keep looking for better answers and keep expecting that surely the medical establishment will change and begin to address this most overwhelming societal and medical disaster. But, as yet, I have seen no evidence of a shift in this direction. I would be delighted to hear, as this book becomes known, of instances where this is not so. But, as of this writing, this seems to be the situation.[2]

Currently, there are many techniques and approaches to recovery that are being tried, and most of them come from the field of alternative medicine, to include Chinese medicine, with its herbs, acupuncture, and ancient understanding of the human subtle energy systems. There is also a lot that has been and is being developed from a more naturopathic approach, focusing largely on supplying the nutritional and supplemental supports that are needed in the recovery process.

There is also a small, and hopefully growing, field of psychiatrists who are called addictionologists. From what I have observed, these are generally M.D.s and psychiatrists who are themselves in recovery, usually of the 12-step and AA variety. The first-person understanding that these physicians bring to their practice is very helpful and much needed. But again, what they've learned about addiction has been largely from their own life stories and from other members of 12-step groups.

Fortunately, these physicians do understand the great care that must be taken in prescribing potentially addictive pharmaceuticals to those who are addicts. Much of the huge influx of addictive substances on the streets, such as oxycodone, is largely due to uninformed physicians prescribing these medications to those who are addicts and know how to manipulate the system. Unscrupulous doctors have also written massive amounts of prescriptions of these controlled substances for profit and, in some cases, individual doctors who have written millions of dollars worth of prescriptions have been arrested, tried, and sentenced. But this is simply the tip of the iceberg and shows a huge systemic problem—partially caused by lack of education and/or a lack of professional ethics.[3]

When searching for alternative treatments (to 12-step models) on the internet, you may feel like you have fallen down the rabbit hole.

You will see acupuncture, animal/pet therapy, aromatherapy, bioelectricity, biofeedback, brainwave biofeedback, creative arts therapy, color therapy, herbal therapy, homeopathy, hypnosis, imagery, journaling, massage, body-work, meditation, spirituality, music, nutrition, qigong, and yoga. (Oy vey!) This is an overwhelming diversity of techniques and approaches, some of which might be very helpful, others of which might not be. I do not believe that any of these holistic treatments, in and of themselves, are a cure for addiction; however, some may be a good nudge in the right direction or helpful in an overall Integral approach. Obviously, we have to evaluate them individually and then determine the best mix of these alternative treatments for our students, collectively and individually.

I do know of two colleagues who are applying the Integral model to the treatment of addiction. My take on them is that they are both extraordinary individuals doing pioneering work. It is certainly to be expected that this list will continue to grow over the next few years.

Guy du Plessis has been working in the field of addiction treatment for over a decade. Since his first encounter with Integral theory, he set out to apply it in the field of addiction treatment and personal recovery. In 2007, as Head of Treatment at Tabankulu Secondary Recovery Centre, in Cape Town, South Africa, he pioneered and implemented an integrally informed clinical in-patient model known as the Integrated Recovery Model (IRM). Since its inception, the model has been implemented in four Cape Town–based treatment centers, and he has trained several addiction counselors in this treatment protocol. He has also pioneered an integrally informed therapy for addicted populations known as Integrated Recovery Therapy, derived from the Integrated Recovery Model. Du Plessis' pioneering work on the IRM has been published in the *Journal of Integral Theory and Practice,* and he is the author of *Integrated Recovery: Recovery in the 21st Century*, currently in review at State University of New York Press.

Ian Waugh is currently director of Bridging the Barriers, a pri-vate counseling, coaching, and training company based on Queensland's Gold Coast, in Australia. Addiction treatment at Bridging the Barriers focuses on empowering people to realize their full potential, strengths, and talents. In 1998, Waugh began to explore how he could develop a holistic approach to addiction treatment. He was introduced to a blend of gestalt therapy and Ken Wilber's Integral model early on, which he continues to use in his work as an addiction therapist. A few years ago, Waugh became interested in incorporating Wilber's Integral Life Practice into his therapeutic work, and at this point he discovered my work and Integral Recovery Practice. Out of our consultations, Waugh developed an out-client's program, which incorporates Integral Recovery Practice and Gestalt Coaching. Waugh says, "The results have been outstanding. I am now using the principles of the Integral Recovery Practice in my consultancy with other treatment services. I am grateful for John's pioneering work."

What I am very sure of at this point is that there is no one silver bullet to kill the dragon of addiction. But I believe that by using the Integral map, we can bring order to this otherwise chaotic and disparate mix. As we learn more about the individual parts, we will have a greater understanding of the big picture. And, as we learn more about the big picture, it will inform us about the usefulness, affordability, and practicality of the individual parts.

It is my hope that the Integral approach will allow us to see how these diverse puzzle pieces fit together in an overall coordinated, ever-evolving, and more effective approach to treatment. I see the Integral approach not as a cure, but as a way to combine the best of what we know so far and begin the work of healing the individual's body, mind, and spirit, as well as our affected culture and political, medical, religious, educational, and law enforcement spheres. All of these are aspects of the whole and have their parts to play. They should begin to work in alignment, as we realize the absolute moral imperative of protecting ourselves, our children, and the generations to come, from what I am now calling the "fifth horseman of the apocalypse."[4] When looked at in an Integral way, we might say that our fifth horseman, addiction, is actually leading the way for the other four—from the gang wars in our streets to the neglect and abuse of children, to the millions of deaths caused by the disease itself and the violence associated with drug trafficking.

Appendix 3

Integral Recovery

An AQAL Approach to Inpatient
Alcohol and Drug Treatment

A Case Study

John Dupuy and Adam Gorman

ABSTRACT This work provides an introduction to the drug and alcohol treatment model Integral Recovery® (IR) developed by John Dupuy.[1] This case study is the first ever written about an integrally informed treatment protocol. A brief introduction to the method is followed by an in depth case study. The IR framework includes the AQAL map and addresses addiction using quadrants, levels, lines, states, and types. This study describes Integral Recovery® in the context of a six-week, residential drug treatment program, in which the recovering addict, Esau, worked individually with John Dupuy, Integral Recovery® founder. The focus of the treatment was on Esau's application of IR concepts and practices to increase the chances of lifelong sobriety and recovery. IR is a scholar-practitioner form of treatment where both the clients and the staff simultaneously engage in practices that foster a community of emotional and spiritual growth.

Alcohol and other mind-altering substances have been around since before recorded history. America's current relationship with drugs is alarming. Califano (2008) notes that although "we have only 4% of the population, we consume over 65% of the worlds drugs. One in four Americans will have an alcohol or drug problem in their lifetime" (Califano, p. xii). Of the large percentage of the population that would qualify for a DSM diagnosis of alcohol and drug dependence, only 10 percent receive treatment. Within this small percentage of the population that is blessed enough to receive a form of inpatient treatment, only 30 percent will successfully remain sober (Califano, p. 69). To put it in another way, only 3 in 10 of all the people currently in treatment for drug and alcohol addiction will remain sober once they leave. The success rates for Alcoholics Anonymous (AA) are equally alarming. A recent study of AA indicates that 60 percent of people who begin attending meetings drop out within the first year (Knack p. 86). This means that a significant portion of people who once sought help with an addiction problem are either attempting to remain sober with no outside help or have relapsed. The authors of this article have deep love for AA and its founders, Bill W. and Dr. Bob. These two men created a free, self-sustaining program that has spread to every continent. The authors, however, propose that more can be done to help the vast majority of people who need treatment and have either not received it, or the treatment they experienced was not sufficient to help them maintain lifelong sobriety.

Integral Recovery was born out of a desire to help the millions of individuals and their loved ones who have not found the help they need from the current recovery programs available. It is our opinion that the application of the AQAL model will lead to increased rates of long-term sobriety among those who employ its practices. The following is a case example from the first ever Integral Recovery (IR) inpatient center. The authors hope to illustrate how the techniques employed by IR will result in greater long-term sobriety for its practitioners.

Integral Theory Applied to Recovery

This section will show how the AQAL map is applied to drug and alcohol treatment.

Integral Recovery® utilizes the comprehensive outlook provided by the AQAL map, applying the four quadrants to address the physical, emotional, spiritual, intellectual, and relational life, including relations with the world—financial, professional, environmental, and technological. Paying equal attention to each of the four quadrants allows for a balanced and effective approach to drug and alcohol treatment.

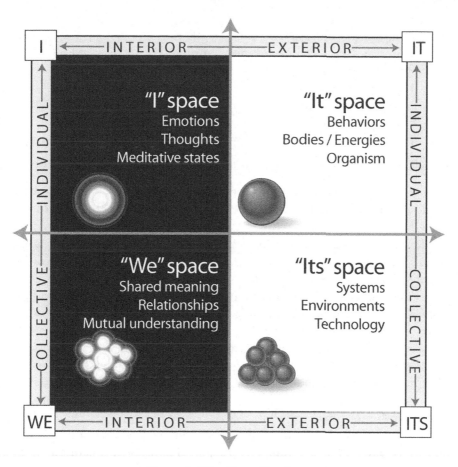

Figure 1. The Four Quadrants

The Upper-Left quadrant represents the interior of the individual. It is the "I" quadrant and encompasses thoughts, feelings, emotions, beliefs, and inner spiritual life (Wilber, p. 62). More than likely, all the activity that has taken place in an addict or alcoholic's Upper-Left quadrant has been geared toward getting drugs or alcohol for some time. He will have many preexisting beliefs about a drug. For example, one belief may be: "I want to quit, but I don't see how I can spend the rest of my life and not use heroin." These thoughts, feelings, beliefs, and, particularly, emotional pain are often acquired during extended use and must be examined in order for the Upper-Left quadrant to become healthy again. In the IR model, we believe it is necessary to go back to the causative factors. If an individual does not evaluate, the contributing Upper-Left causes such as loneliness, isolation, lack of meaning/purpose, the chances of long-term sobriety will be reduced.

Esau's Upper-Left quadrant was stable when he arrived in Utah. What was obvious from the outset was what an excellent attitude he had. His demeanor was one of commitment and genuine gratitude for the opportunity to get sober. He was, however, mentally exhausted and experiencing noticeable anxiety. What arose over the first few days was Esau's anger at himself for relapsing, as well as his sense of missed opportunity. He was very judgmental of himself for falling back into drug addiction again. What also became evident in the first week of treatment was that Esau was not comfortable going into his emotional pain. This made sense considering Esau's Enneagram type, a Seven, which typically avoids painful emotional exploration. The use of the Enneagram will be discussed later in this case study.

The Upper-Right quadrant represents the exterior of the individual. This is the quadrant of "It," meaning the body: circulatory system, muscles, brain chemistry, bones, etc. (Wilber p. 63). This aspect of a person can be seen, touched, and measured. Often, when someone enters treatment, he has been neglecting and damaging his body for a while. Extensive drug and alcohol use takes a vast toll on the body, and the physical side effects of prolonged use must be addressed as part of an Integral Recovery® program.

Esau's Upper-Right quadrant needed immediate attention. He was exhausted and was having difficulty sleeping. He had lost 20 pounds since his relapse began and was underweight. An addiction to cigarettes was also interfering with his health. He had already detoxed from heroin, and there were no remaining physical signs of addiction. He was placed on a regimen of multivitamins, protein, and fish oil. The food he ate was all organic and designed to replenish his body with the nutrients it had not received while he was using heroin and cocaine.

The Lower-Left quadrant is the "We" space, or plural interiors, the collective subjective dimension (Wilber p. 63). In any individual, there are things occurring in both the interior and exterior at all times. The Lower-Left quadrant deals with the collective interiors, such as family and romantic relationships. It also includes healthy community support, such as a church or a sobriety support group like AA. The Lower-Left quadrant factors greatly into the treatment of addiction, as most often addicts enter recovery having damaged or destroyed many of the relationships they claim to cherish the most. Often, an alcoholic will enter treatment because of an ultimatum given by his or her family or significant other.

Esau's Lower-Left quadrant was in a state of tension. His family was angry and hurt over his behavior. He had just begun to reestablish a relationship with his teenage daughter after a long separation, but this ended when he relapsed. His son was living with Esau's parents, and Esau was an active part of his life before he needed to enter treatment again. All of these strained family relations spilled over from Esau's Lower-Left to his Upper-Left quadrant in the form of anger and a poor self-image. This is an excellent example of struggle in one quadrant affecting the harmony of the other three.

John Dupuy made weekly telephone calls to Esau's family and gave them assignments to better understand the disease of addiction and the way it affects the brain. These assignments centered around the work of Dr. Kevin McCauley and his work on the disease model of addiction. John also recommended to the family members that they start using binaural brainwave entrainment (BBE) meditation and encouraged them to attend regular Al Anon meetings. The family component of IR will be discussed later in this study.

The Lower-Right quadrant is the "Its" space. This represents the plural exteriors of an individual (Wilber p. 63). It includes the external world: nature, the internet, highways, the economy, the entire web of life. It also includes employment, school, insurance, or involvement with the legal system, to name a few. Being in active addiction is a full-time job, and individuals who enter recovery have often depleted their financial resources. It is also not uncommon for people new to recovery to be facing legal charges as a result of their use. IR takes all of these Lower-Right possibilities into account when formulating a unique treatment plan by taking an in-depth inventory as part of the intake process.

Esau's Lower-Right quadrant had taken a significant hit during his relapse. Esau entered IR with no observable physical or psychological disabilities besides addiction. During his time on the street, Esau had gone through $30,000 dollars in savings. He had lost his house and was relying on his parents to support him financially. This Lower-Right quadrant dependence on his parents produced a sense of shame and failure in Esau's Upper-Left quadrant, which, like the effects of the strained relationships in the Lower-Left quadrant, spilled into Esau's Upper-Left interiors. It was discovered that underneath Esau's shame at needing to be supported, there were underlying feelings of sadness and anger about never being able to live up to his father's expectations. These themes continued to arise in various forms throughout Esau's time in treatment.

The disease of addiction affects all four quadrants. The Upper-Right quadrant has to contend with the brain disease of addiction and the way it depletes both brain chemistry and body of essential nourishing elements; in the Upper-Left quadrant, the disease causes emotional and spiritual pain and cognitive impairment that accumulate over extended use; in the Lower-Left quadrant, addiction creates a cultural and interpersonal strain on relationships and loved ones; and in the Lower-Right quadrant, it is a social disease that reveals itself in homelessness, violence, and drunk driving, to name a few.

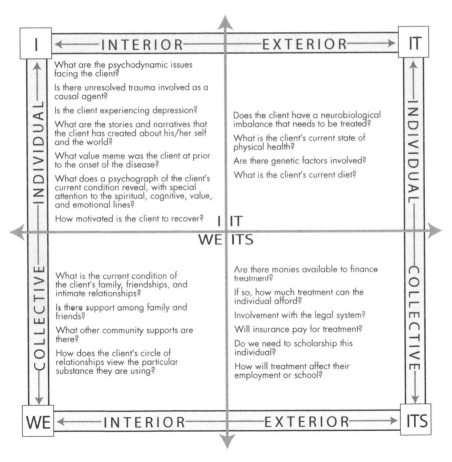

Figure 2. Four-Quadrant Treatment Assessment

Stages

By using the AQAL map, Integral Recovery incorporates developmental levels into the process of recovery. By incorporating Spiral Dynamics (Beck, 1996), Integral Recovery® is able to provide much more comprehensive, individualized treatment plans than traditional treatment. Every client has unique needs based on his developmental level. For example, someone who is at the orange modern/rationalist level will have very different motivations for sobriety than someone at the green postmodern/ pluralistic level. IR designs a unique treatment program that will resonate for each level's perspective and needs.

Esau arrived at treatment at a green meme center of gravity. His center of gravity was based on the professional judgment and experience of John Dupuy. However, because of his consistent drug use, he had regressed to an egocentric level of moral development despite having reached a worldcentric level during his previous period of sobriety. It is common for addicts to enter treatment at an egocentric moral level. Esau's motivations to come to Integral Recovery were green to Integral; however, his behaviors as he was acting out addiction were red, based in part on the increased activation of the midbrain that occurs during active use. The lifestyle of addiction demands this regression in order to justify the behavior often required to obtain drugs or alcohol. We have found after years of clinical experience that most people return to their preaddiction moral level of development after their use has stopped. The regression that takes place during relapse and active addiction is an area that has great potential for further research.

After his return to the worldcentric level, Esau was given readings that would foster his love and knowledge of Integral. He was able to read, comprehend, and internalize many writings of Ken Wilber. A large part of his treatment was processing these readings on an emotional level and not just in the mental realm where Esau was most comfortable. He was also very blessed to spend a significant amount of time with Diane Hamilton and Roland Stanich, who were staying nearby. These interactions with leading Integral thinkers certainly were inspiring for Esau.

States

States are the basic dimensions of human consciousness: waking, dreaming, and deep sleep (Wilber, p. 12). Meditative and spiritual experiences are also states. Anything that arises in an individual's awareness, including thoughts, feelings, and experiences is considered a state. IR begins teaching its students early on to identify the gross, subtle, causal, and nondual states that arise in them phenomenologically. A major presenting problem with addicts and alcoholics is that they want to hold onto the positive states and avoid the negative ones. This tendency is especially evident with people who are Sevens on the Enneagram, like Esau.

Esau already had an advanced working knowledge of states. Although he had extensive cognitive knowledge of states, he avoided experiencing many of those he classified as negative. Because of his past avoidance and its link to relapse, it was essential for Esau to begin to accept all of his emotions and not just the positive ones. He began listening to BBE audio tracks for a minimum of two hours a day and worked on accepting, observing, and releasing any emotions that arose during his sessions. John Dupuy offered assistance and guidance throughout this process because much of what arose was painful and required the presence of a skilled guide. Through meditation, shadow and trauma work, and employing the Sedona Method and 3-2-1 techniques adapted by Dupuy for the process of Integral Recovery, Esau began to approach the processing and release of negative emotions as a fundamental component of his IR plan.

Lines

Integral Recovery® draws on the work of Ken Wilber and Howard Gardner and his theory of Multiple Intelligences (Gardner, 1993). Lines are semi-independent capacities that vary in development depending upon the individual. These include cognitive intelligence, spiritual intelligence, emotional intelligence, kinesthetic intelligence. Rather than referring to these individual measures collectively as intelligence, IR borrows from the work of Gardner and calls them lines. Distinguishing between the multiple components of intelligence enables the measuring of one against another. For example, someone could be highly developed spiritually but lack emotional intelligence. If an individual is highly developed in one line but stagnant in another, then he is out of balance and will eventually run into trouble. The five main lines that IR concentrates on (although there are many more) are (1) spiritual, (2) emotional, (3) cognitive, (4) physical, and (5) ethical. Like all IR clients, Esau had the location of his lines assessed during his initial AQAL assessment so that an individualized treatment plan could be developed for him. At this point, this assessment is largely intuitive in the spiritual, emotional, and cognitive lines; in the physical line, there are tests that measure neurochemical balances. In Esau's case, these tests were prohibitively expensive.

Spiritual

Esau has been a Christian all his life and is interested in the work of contemplative Christianity. A priest introduced him to the work of Ken Wilber, so the components of an Integral lifestyle were already linked at some level to his spiritual faith.

Esau meditated a minimum of one hour in the morning and one hour in the afternoon, using BBE. During this time, he incorporated prayer and contemplation to combine his spiritual faith with the benefits of BBE meditation.

Emotional

Esau has a life history of being emotionally avoidant. One of the negative behaviors of a Seven on the Enneagram is the tendency to avoid (Riso et al., p. 263). Over time, these feelings built up and contributed to his drug use and relapses. A large part of Esau's work with John was to become comfortable recognizing and accepting unwanted feelings and shadow. Learning effective coping skills is essential if Esau is to avoid relapse when he leaves treatment. Learning to work with states as they arise and hold them in an open awareness that is beyond states is what is referred to as the "science of happiness" in Integral parlance as we learn to be present and accept whatever emotional states arise.

Cognitive

Esau was highly advanced cognitively. He entered IR with an extensive knowledge of Integral theory. This helped tremendously because normally someone in early recovery will need to be introduced to the AQAL map and learn the basic theory. In Esau's case, he was able to jump right in and start the second phase of the work.

Physical

As described earlier, Esau was experiencing anxiety and difficulty sleeping. He was underweight and had not had a consistent exercise practice for some time. Upon arrival in treatment, Esau began practicing yoga on a daily basis and strength training six days a week. He also began running, and eventually he was able to run 10 miles with relative ease.

Type

In deference to the insight of Ken Wilber in including typologies as an essential part of the AQAL map, the Enneagram in particular has proved to be a very powerful part of the IR model. Types are the basic personality styles or orientations, such as masculine/feminine, sexual and cultural, and personality types as represented by the Enneagram. This form of typology provides an imminently useful and compelling "sacred psychology" that facilitates psychological healing and growth as well as spiritual awakening. Being able to differentiate masculine and feminine as well as Enneagram types is crucial to an Integral Recovery® program. The needs of a Five are very different from the needs of an Eight, when it comes to therapy and the healing of past wounds. It is not uncommon for an addiction counselor to believe something that worked for himself personally should and will work for everyone in the same way. This one-size-fits-all approach can result in many people who are in drug and alcohol treatment never receiving the individualized treatment they need

A major shortcoming of mainstream recovery programs is that they often approach every individual in the same way and, as a result, overlook some crucial needs of early recovery. IR takes into account both the horizontal type of the Enneagram and the vertical level of development on the spiral dynamic scale. IR definitely includes other developmental models (e.g., Ken Wilber's model and the model of Susanne Cook-Greuter); we start, however, with Spiral Dynamics, as it is accessible and immediately useful in helping clients see themselves and their world with new eyes.

Esau is a Seven on the Enneagram. Sevens at their best are "opti-mistic, enthusiastic, curious, entrepreneurial, imaginative, spontaneous, productive, fun-loving, charming, and confident." At their worst, they are "rebellious, thrill seeking, narcissistic, scattered, uncommitted, undisciplined, impulsive, self-destructive, manic, over-talkative, and insensitive" (Riso et al., p. 279). Sevens often avoid pain by staying busy and never sitting with their emotions. It is not uncommon for a Seven to have to work hard to move below surface level. Esau displayed the Seven's tendency of emotional avoidance, and he was also largely unaware of his emotions and feelings. As described earlier, BBE and emotional releasing work, along with shadow work facilitated by John Dupuy, were the primary interventions to Esau's avoidance. Esau was well versed in Integral theory and quickly became fully committed to his regimen of shadow exploration and release.

Treatment

Esau first contacted me via e-mail.[2] He said he had discovered my website and that he was convinced that this was the model for him. I called Esau, and he informed me that he had been struggling with drug addiction since his mid-teens. At this time he was thirty-one years old. He said he was addicted primarily to cocaine and heroin and had a history of heavy drug use interspersed with treatment and some sobriety followed by relapse. Esau said he was desperate to stop using and wanted my help.

Esau informed me that he was a fan of Ken Wilber and Integral theory. I told him I did not have a treatment center at the time, but his earnestness convinced me that perhaps we could work together one on one. We made arrangements for Esau to fly to Utah, and I picked him up early in the morning at a motel in Salt Lake City four days after our initial contact.

Esau appeared to be very grateful, somewhat anxious, and eager to get to work. After initially checking in, we went to Whole Foods to stock up on the necessary supplements and lots of healthy, organic food. Then, as I am wont to do with new students, I had Esau begin his practices on the three and a half hour-long drive back to my home in Southern Utah. He started his supplements and began doing cranial electrical stimulation and BBE meditation as we drove. Esau already had some experience using BBE (which he had used sporadically). This set the tone for the rest of our time together: practice, practice, practice.

The next six weeks were characterized by the following daily routine. It should be noted that Esau was already familiar with the AQAL map and Integral language.

Daily Routine

We would wake up at six o'clock (approximately), meet in the kitchen, and Esau would prepare organic juice with a juicer, which we would drink together. We would then do a 20-minute yoga routine, using a video produced by Gaiam, featuring Rodney Yee. After yoga, we would do an hour of BBE meditation. I let Esau have a pen and paper while he meditated in order to jot down significant things that would come up during the meditation. Using BBE, this seems to work very well to capture insights, so they can be verbally worked later and does not take away from the deep work that this type of meditation makes possible. After meditation, I would give Esau a few minutes to journal his experience, and then we would discuss what had come up. This provided for a very powerful one-on-one counseling period. I would use an eclectic blend of psychotherapeutic approaches, most notably motivational interviewing (Miller p. 23).

After meditation, journaling, and counseling, we would eat breakfast. After breakfast, we would work on the cognitive line: teachings, readings, and listening to talks and CDs as was appropriate for where Esau was at in the treatment process. (I had sent Esau the as yet unpublished manuscript of my book, *Integral Recovery*, after our first phone conversation, which he then read in two days. This set a great tone and gave him a good understanding of the work we would be doing together before he even arrived; it allowed us to cut directly to the chase.)

In the first couple of days, I had Esau listen to *The Disease Model of Addiction,* by Kevin McCauley, M.D. In this CD, Dr. McCauley elegantly and clearly explains that addiction is a brain disease and not a result of character flaws, sin, or addictive personalities. (I now use the very good Dr. Kevin McCauley DVD *Pleasure Unwoven.*) I cover this material extensively in my writings, but I feel Dr. McCauley's introduction is a great help. I find this information to be very revelatory and useful, not only for addicts, but also for their families and loved ones. I had Esau listen to this material and take notes, and then we would discuss it. One of my guiding principles in teaching is that repetition is the law of memory, so I hammer home the basics and get my students to teach them back to me.

After the morning cognitive work, we would go to the gym and start Esau on his rigorous strength-training routine. It might be noted that Esau was very enthusiastic in the gym, and I had a hard time holding him back from pushing himself too hard initially. Interestingly enough, I find this is true with most of my students.

After lunch, which, as with all of our meals, was always healthy and organic, Esau would have a break until our afternoon/evening meditation session. During this time, which was normally about three and a half hours, Esau could take a nap, go for a walk, or work on the reading or written assignments that he was given (see reading list). This would also give me time to catch up on my work, writing, and other clients. Around 4:30 p.m., we would do another hour of BBE meditation followed by journaling and process work. We would then prepare and eat dinner together, often with my wife and other members of our community, and then have the rest of the evening off for taking walks, resting, reading, working on assignments, and so on.

The idea that has emerged from my work with clients is that we practice hard and also have a lot of time to rest, recreate, and recuperate. This was our day-to-day pattern and flow. In addition to this, once a week we would wake up early and head to a trail near my house called Velvet Ridge and do a 10-mile run. As this was usually very early, Esau and I would often do our BBE meditation as we jogged. This became a beloved part of our work together. It also became a beautiful metaphor for the long, lifetime journey of recovery and growth.

On weekends, we would often take trips out into the wilderness where we would continue our meditation and work, but in a context of adventure and exploration of the beautiful Wayne County wilderness. On Sunday mornings, Esau would participate in our weekly meditation group, which has been meeting every Sunday morning in our home for approximately 14 years.

Esau was also able to go to Diane Hamilton's Boulder Mountain Zen Center to meditate, which is located about three miles from my house. He could do this in the evenings, but only if he had completed his two hours of BBE meditation. This became one of our running jokes: the reward for meditation is more meditation.

One of the advantages of the Integral approach to addiction is that one learns to speak about treatment in terms that reflect the client's spiritual traditions and development level. In Esau's case, it emerged that Esau is a devout Christian of the Catholic persuasion, and we were able to discuss our spiritual practice and work in terms of the Christian tradition and contemplative meditation and prayer. When I work with a group of students, this can, at times, be a little more challenging, but in Esau's case, it was very easy as I also come from the same background and could work with him on an individual basis.

Vision Quest

During the first week of Esau's treatment, I spoke with him a little about my own vision-questing experience. Esau immediately grabbed onto this idea as something he wanted to do while he was with me. So we scheduled a vision quest for him during his fourth week of treatment. I have a lot of experience using vision questing as part of treatment. Esau asked me if he could bring his BBE track with him on his iPod, and after some reflection, I said yes. This turned out to be very powerful and successful in Esau's case. I initially felt some consternation about this as it didn't seem very traditional; then I asked myself exactly which tradition was I protecting, and the answer was—none.

During the fourth week, Esau did a four-day, three-night vision quest in the National Forest bordering Wayne County. A vision quest is modeled after the Native American rite-of-passage ceremony. It should be noted that a vision quest is not a necessary part of an Integral Recovery program, but wilderness therapy is an excellent complement to primary treatment. Esau was very enthusiastic at the start of his vision quest and spent the majority of his first day using BBE. Toward the end of the day, he fell asleep and slept until early afternoon of the following day. He awoke frustrated at himself for not being more disciplined. His thoughts began to spiral, and by midday he was questioning his ability to complete the vision quest. At that point, he began using BBE, and he recalls "breaking through a wall and experiencing a feeling of intense peace and contentment wash over me." As the day progressed, Esau reported a feeling of immense unity with all things, particularly with the animals that visited him in his campsite. He said that he experienced "the connection that he longed for while doing drugs." This feeling remained with him throughout the following days. When asked what he had gained from his vision quest, he said, "I feel like my vision quest was when all the separate strands of insight that I had gained from my time with John became glued together. Before, the knowledge was just in my mind, but I came back with wisdom inside of me."

Family Weekend

During the fifth week of treatment, Esau's parents, brother, and six-year-old son came to Wayne County for the family portion of treatment. It should be noted that I had weekly phone conversations on Sunday evenings with Esau's parents to keep them informed of what was going on and also to recommend readings, Dr. McCauley's DVD, and recommend that they get started on their own binaural brainwave entrainment meditation programs.

The family portion of Esau's treatment went as follows. On the first morning, I allowed Esau to spend time with his son, while I discussed the basics of Integral Recovery and addiction with Esau's family. After that, Esau described to his family what he had learned throughout his treatment. In the afternoon, we did the four R's: Resentments, Regrets, Respects, and Requests. These are lists that I told both Esau and his adult family members to prepare before they arrived at my home.

In resentments, each member prepared a list of the things that they resent the other person doing to their relationship. For example, Esau's father might have written something like this: "Esau, I resent that you stole so much from me to buy your drugs." After listing their resentments, each person would write their regrets—things they regretted having done to their relationship. For example, Esau might write, "Dad, I regret that I stole money from you so often in order to buy drugs."

In the respects column, you list the things you respect about the other person. For example, Esau might have written, "Dad, I respect how hard you worked to support our family." And the last category, requests, consists of requests that each individual makes to the other. For example, Esau's mother might have written, "Esau, I request that you stay faithful to your daily Integral Recovery practices."

How all of this looks in practice is that Esau and his father would sit in straight-backed chairs facing each other, knee to knee, a few inches apart, and Esau would start with his 4 Rs list. While each person can read from his list, they are instructed to maintain eye contact, and the other person is instructed to reflect back (not interpret) what the other has said. For example, Esau might have said, "Dad, I resent that you were never around very much when I was growing up." And the father would respond, "I hear that you resent that I was not around very much when you were growing up." This is done slowly and deliberately, and I (along with my wife, Pam, who is an excellent therapist) was there to offer suggestions and coaching if necessary. This is an amazingly powerful process, which I have used hundreds of times with many families. It seems to be very cathartic and clears the air of all the lurking elephants in the room.

The next day, we worked on relapse prevention, relapse plans—what happens if I do relapse, or if you relapse—and warning signs (behaviors that Esau's family could observe that would be warning signs that perhaps relapse had occurred or might be imminent). We also discussed triggers: people, places, and things that could put Esau at risk, such as old playmates and old playgrounds that Esau frequented when he was using. And we discussed the logistics of what would be the followup after Esau left treatment with me, such as continuing his practices, getting a therapist, doing couples counseling with his girlfriend, family counseling, and weekly coaching calls with me. All of this was a very powerful process with much healing and gratitude expressed on all sides.

After Esau's family left, we continued with our final week of work together. After our six weeks together, Esau found a local motel, where he stayed to attend an Integral Zen workshop with Diane Hamilton. It also might be noted that during this period we took field trips to Salt Lake City and Boulder, Colorado, where Esau was able to meet and spend time with most of his Integral heroes, for example, Ken Wilber, Diane Hamilton, Rollie Stanich, and Rob McNamara. It should be noted that these interactions were unique and are not considered standard for an IR residential. They certainly enhanced Esau's experience.

The Developmental Dimension

In my earlier writings, I have talked a lot about how the developmental dimension of the AQAL map lends itself so brilliantly to the process of recovery by deepening our understanding of the dynamics of the recovery process.

In Esau's recovery, however, a dynamic emerged that covered new ground. One of the elements of Esau's drug history was the fact that he managed, at various times, to have a period of sobriety punctuated and ended by relapse. Esau's sober developmental level seemed to be a rather enthusiastic green meme and a Seven on the Enneagram. However, when Esau would relapse, his green level of development would almost immediately slide back to a toxic, egocentric red stage, in which his former kindness and concern for others would change into the Mr. Hyde, sociopathic manipulator. While Esau was using drugs, all his relationships were either neglected or manipulated in order to secure more drugs. At the same time, Esau somewhat maintained a green exterior, but his motivations were definitely egocentric and red. The decision to start using drugs again is propelled by the reptilian brainstem and not the higher values associated with the neocortex (McCauley audio CD). This activation of survival instincts is responsible for the rapid descent from green to red value memes.

I have heard this condition referred to by some as being a water-melon: green on the outside, red on the inside. So what we see here is a vast fluctuation in the developmental center of gravity, depending on whether Esau was sober or not, which confirms my anecdotal observations that the highest former, predrug level of moral development can quickly be regained when the recovery process is actively engaged. The AQAL map is hugely valuable for increasing understanding of this aspect of addiction and the self-knowledge that the recovering addict acquires from this understanding. This becomes a motivational imperative for continuing Integral Recovery Practice and sobriety. Do I want to live for my highest potential or live from my most abased and degraded self.

Component Parts of the Integral Recovery Treatment Program

1. Brainwave Entrainment Meditation

I have been using BWE meditation for over seven years in my own practice and with my clients. Brainwave entrainment is a technology that uses sound listened to through stereo headphones to put the user into very deep, meditational states. In addition to being pleasant, therefore doable—unlike unassisted normal meditation—users begin to experience the fruits of a deep, healing, disciplined meditation practice almost immediately (Harris 2007). In a recent study by Wahbeh, binaural beat technology was shown to decrease anxiety and increase quality of life measurements (Wahbeh et al., p. 1). Having tried normal meditation, or unassisted, traditional meditation, with recovering addicts for many years, the use of BWE meditation is truly a quantum leap forward in the treatment field in the following areas:

1. Spirituality truly becomes an injunction, a practice that one does to begin to discover one's own essential truth, as opposed to the traditional more dogmatic approach, "You need to believe this." In Integral Recovery, you do the injunction, in this case the Profound Meditation Program (PMP), and your beliefs emerge from your own internal experiences.

2. Shadow work. With PMP and supportive instructions, clients are soon able to confront, transform, and transmute their own shadow issues. Again, this is a quantum leap forward in the

field of recovery. One of the primary causes of serial relapse for addicts who have been in treatment is the fact that they were never able to deal with their past traumas, current stress, and shadow material. Traditionally, group therapy and individual therapy have been used to attempt to deal with these issues, and, too often, they do not work.

3. Brain healing and transformation. PMP begins to synchronize the left and right hemispheres of the brain and to rebalance the brain neurochemically, increasing the levels of healthy neurochemicals that have been depleted through the use of drugs and alcohol, such as serotonin and dopamine, and decreasing the negative, stress-related neurochemicals, such as CRF and cortisol (Harris, p. 8).

4. In my work with addicts, I have found that very soon into their PMP process, they begin to have deep insights into the nature of their personal conflicts and subsequent disease. This is very powerful, as almost always the truth that comes out of *your* mouth about *you* is more powerful than the truth that comes out of *my* mouth about you. They begin to wake up.

5. Increased intelligence. Very quickly in the process of brain-wave entrainment meditation, I have noticed time and again that mental functioning increases. In other words, recovering addicts actually begin to understand what the hell Ken Wilber, I, and other Integral teachers are talking about.

2. The Enneagram

I have found that using the Enneagram with my students is a very powerful, even essential, part of Integral Recovery. The Enneagram truly provides a "sacred psychology" that helps my students understand their own ego traps and see the path that they must take to become whole and healthy. Traditionally, one is supposed to let the student figure out for herself what type she is on the Enneagram; however, often it is very clear to me, and I will simply tell her, explain the basics, and then have her read about her type. In Esau's case, it was a revelation to him. It would not be too much to say that "the scales fell from his eyes." Esau began to understand his patterns, why he used drugs, and what could lead him to relapse. These insights became an integral part of our daily conversations and work together.

3. Cranial Electrical Stimulation (CES)

CES is a technology that has been around since the first decade of the twentieth century, and its efficacy has been proven in clinical studies in the United States, Europe, and Russia. It is approved by the FDA in this country and emits a low electrical current to stimulate the brain. IR uses the CES Stimulator manufactured by Fisher Wallace. The electrical current is delivered by damp sponges that are placed on the temples and held in place by a headband. The Stimulator uses two AA batteries and is adjusted by the individual so he can feel a slight tingling sensation. What this does is rebalance the neurochemistry of the brain to an optimal level in very short order (Mellen et al., p. 14). One of the problems in early recovery, and one that often leads to relapse, is that the brain of the addict has been gravely depleted of essential neurochemicals. This leads to a condition called anhedonia, in which the addict is unable to experience pleasure from normal, healthy activities and can only experience pleasure from using substances (Hutchison p. 315).

CES almost immediately begins to restore optimal chemical balance in the brain (Hutchison p. 315). We use this along with PMP meditation: headphones and ear clips. Often my clients have said that using CES at the same time deepens their meditation. CES has also been used extensively to treat clinical depression and sleep disorders (Hutchison p. 315). I have found this to be a very powerful and quick way to restore mental health and to facilitate positive personality changes while working with my clients.

4. Nutritional Supplements

Esau's daily supplements consisted of the following:

1. 5-HTP, an amino acid that is a precursor to serotonin and has been effective in increasing available serotonin levels in the brain.

2. A vitamin/mineral supplement. Esau used one called Vitamin Code for Men. This is a vitamin and mineral supplement that

uses a technology that attaches the nutritional supplements to food molecules to make them more available and absorbable to the body than normal supplements.

3.   A high-grade purified fish oil supplement that supplies essential fatty acids to help rebuild and stabilize brain health and functioning.

4.   A powerful phytonutrient such as spirulina or chlorella to provide phytonutrients from plant sources.

5.   A general amino acid supplement that includes all the major essential and nonessential amino acids.

6.   Kudzu, an extract that has been used in Chinese medicine for centuries to decrease cravings for alcohol.

5. Yoga

I need to say a little about the benefits of yoga because in our Integral Recovery Practice, we use yoga, cardio, and strength training, as well as diet and supplementation, as the pillars of our healthy body line. I have found that a morning yoga routine is very helpful in getting us prepared for our morning meditation, as well as keeping us limber and increasing a sense of well-being throughout the day.

6. Strength Training with Mindfulness

I taught Esau strength training, which involves using free weights and machines, very much influenced by the work of Shawn Phillips and Rob McNamara. We would also use our time in the gym as a time to practice mindfulness, by using intense focus as we worked each muscle group. We would also pause in my car, before going into the gym, for a few moments of silent prayer in which we would dedicate our practice to the highest good that we were capable of imagining that day (e.g., to God, my sobriety, my family, all sentient beings, generations to come, etc.).

7. Written Exercises

I gave Esau various written assignments, such as answering the question "What are the impediments that keep you from practicing and maintaining your sobriety?" I also had him write out his life history and drug history and share it with me. These assignments can be completely individualized for each client's needs.

8. Reading List

I assigned Esau the following books to read. The reading list is unique to each client and centered around his specific needs.

> *Everything Belongs,* by Richard Rohr.
> *High Society: How Substance Abuse Ravages America and What We Can Do About It,* by Joseph A. Califano.
> *Integral Psychology,* by Ken Wilber.
> *Translucent Revolution: How People Like You Are Waking Up and Changing the World,* by Arjuna Ardagh.
> *The Way of the Superior Man,* by David Deida.
> *The Wisdom of the Enneagram,* by Don Richard Riso and Russ Hudson.

9. Family Profound Meditation Program Meditation

I had Esau's family do BWE meditation, and we meditated together during the family treatment process.

10. Community Participation

The opportunity for Esau to participate in our community, which is by and large spiritual, holistic, very loving, and increasingly Integral, was a major eye opener for him. Comparing this experience with that of hanging out with the people he had been with before was like night and day for Esau.

Progress during Treatment

Esau's progress during treatment was very dramatic. When he first arrived, his appearance was beaten down, exhausted, and somewhat emaciated. While Esau's attitude was very positive, he exhibited a great deal of anxiety and underlying feelings of shame and hopelessness. During treatment, his physical vitality returned very quickly, and remarkably, he began to express a deep sense of connected spirituality within the first few days.

Esau's root tradition is Roman Catholic Christianity. In fact, the first person to introduce him to the works of Ken Wilber was an enlightened priest at his local church. John Dupuy also comes from a Catholic Christian background; his initial spiritual opening was of a Christian variety, and this part of him has deepened as his Integral practice has deepened. Therefore, working with Esau one on one, it was possible to speak of the work in terms of Christian contemplative practice, using scripture, praying together, and talking about meditation and contemplation in Christian mystical terms. Richard Rohr's book, *Everything Belongs*, was one of the key texts used during treatment. This is a beautiful example of how Integral Recovery can work with people where they are at and in language that is understandable to them. Contemplative Christianity has great depth, richness, and strength to add to the Integral Recovery journey for those who are open to it.

There were two occasions in which Esau's Mr. Hyde personality surfaced. Once on a long run and once when he wanted to drop everything and go to a Rainbow Gathering. The fact that this subpersonality surfaced was frankly a relief to John, as it offered an opportunity for Esau and John to look together at the anger and the "fuck you" attitude that is part and parcel of the addictive personality.

At one point during treatment, Esau really got the message, "It's not all about me." The teaching became very clear that before acting impulsively, or thinking, "This is what I want and I want it now," it's important to think about other perspectives (i.e., that of Esau's parents, his children, his future, God's will, etc.). Esau was able to hear this, and for lack of a better term became truly repentant and changed his attitude. At times, John and Esau would actually hug each other and cry together. This gives an idea of the intimacy of working with someone so closely day in and day out for six weeks.

Again, the vehicle for Esau and other recovery addicts' continued sobriety and growth is the Integral Recovery Practice itself. Once Esau became dedicated to and firmly established in his practices, he became more independent and more responsible for his own recovery process. This is exactly what John had in mind when he first envisioned Integral Recovery.

By the time Esau's parents were due to arrive, Esau was anxious about seeing them and hoping very much that they would be able to understand the progress he had made and that they would support his work. During the family weekend, Esau's younger brother showed up unexpectedly, as well as his six-year-old son and his parents. The weekend was very profound and healing. Esau's family was definitely a "good enough" family with strong resources both emotionally and financially.

By the last week of treatment, Esau had come to the point where he was very established in his practices and was preparing to do a 10-day Integral Zen Intensive with Integral Recovery's friend, colleague, and neighbor Diane Musho Hamilton. John felt that this was an important aspect of treatment in that it not only reinforced Esau's practices, but also gave him Lower-Left support as he was able to hang out with a large group of amazing Integral people.

After Esau's six-week stay was up, John continued working with him on Skype. Esau progressed steadily and was able to set up support systems consisting primarily of his family and his Zen teacher in his hometown, as well as connecting with a very powerful Integral practice group. One of the challenges that Esau faced soon after returning home was a rather nasty breakup with his girlfriend. Esau was able to handle this quite well, which was very important because problems with the same person had led to his last relapse.

One of the truisms of Integral Recovery is that during stressful times we increase our practices. Often people will say, "Oh, there is so much going on. I don't have time to practice now." But in IR, we increase our time and dedication to our practices during difficult times: instead of doing PMP for an hour a day, we might do it for one and a half or two hours. (In treatment, which serves as IR boot camp, we meditate a minimum of two hours a day; however, when one returns to the world, the requirement is only one hour a day, or more depending on one's personal needs.)

Two-Month Check-in (A Two-Month Follow-up Conversation with Esau)

I contacted Esau by phone two months after he returned to the Midwest to ask him what his general impressions were of Integral Recovery. He was living at his parent's house and being financially supported by them. He said the entire experience was amazing, from the organic food and daily workouts to his vision quest and individual sessions with John. Esau also felt his Integral Recovery experience was heightened by the opportunity to spend time with Integral thinkers like Diane Hamilton and

Roland Stanich. I asked if there was a piece of the program that stood out more than any other. He told me that Integral Recovery's emphasis on practice and extensive shadow work is what enabled him to gain as much as he did from his time in Utah. I inquired why this part of the program stood out to him, and he explained that his previous attempts at recovery had been decent efforts, but he never did the necessary shadow work. Esau said that his use of BBE meditation followed by his one-on-one shadow work sessions enabled him to go into his pain in a much deeper way than he had previously.

The conversation then shifted to how he has maintained his Integral Recovery Practice since his return to the Midwest. Esau has maintained his sobriety despite the deaths of three of his close friends within a two-month period of time. He also broke up with his girlfriend, so he could fully devote himself to his own sobriety; he explained that his practice is the number one priority in his life. He continues to use BBE on a daily basis and has joined a gym and a Zen center. Most important, Esau states that when his pain and shadow arise, he does not avoid them. He views avoidance as starting off down the road of relapse.

Toward the end of our conversation, I asked Esau if there was anything in particular that he has realized since he left that was important to mention. He said, "I used to view practice as physical or mental activity that made you feel good, but now I think of it as the glue of my sobriety. Without my practice, I would lose all the momentum I have gained over the past few months."

Six-Month Check-in

After six months of continuous sobriety, Esau returned to Wayne County, Utah, to work as John's assistant. Recently Esau has taken over supervision of the daily activities including BWE meditation, yoga, and visits to the gym. He continues to engage in all the practices and is using his past experience to educate and inspire the next generation of IR students.

Postscript

As I am preparing the final edits to this book, Esau passed his two-year sobriety birthday. He is currently enrolled in a university and has completed his first semester. He has continued his Integral Recovery practices and has expressed to me that some of his greatest current challenges are simply adjusting to being "back in the world"—paying the bills and taking care of the day-to-day Lower-Right quadrant issues that he never dealt with during his long drug-taking career. Esau is also working on his relationship with his parents and his son, who currently lives with his parents. Instead of running from these responsibilities and relationships, Esau is now facing them.

Conclusion

The success of IR is a result of how it transcends and includes other recovery programs. IR makes use of recent scientific breakthroughs and research that were unavailable to other recovery organizations when they were being formed. As a result, these authors believe the additional treatment components that an Integral approach contributes are the next evolutionary steps in a field with overall low long-term success rates. Preliminary client outcome results have been promising and indicate high success rates in the first five years since IR has been operating. Additional long-term studies are required to substantiate these early findings, but preliminary results indicate success rates one-third more successful than the country's leading treatment facilities.

Based on these preliminary findings, these authors believe that Integral Recovery promises to be a much more effective treatment model for the disease of addiction. The use of the AQAL model provides a much more comprehensive approach to the disease of addiction than formerly available. The combination of brainwave entrainment technology, cranial electrical stimulation, a highly regimented Integral Life Plan, and intensive shadow work has shown, in preliminary case studies, to drastically increase the chances of long-term sobriety.

Case Study References

Beck, D. E., and Cowan, C. C. *Spiral Dynamics: Mastering Values, Leadership, and Change.* Blackwell Publishers, 1996.

Califano, J. *High Society: How Substance Abuse Ravishes America and What to Do About It.* New York: Public Affairs™, a member of the Perseus Books Group, 2008.

Gardner, Howard. *Frames of Mind: The Theory of Multiple Intelligences.* New York: Basic Books, 1993.

Harris, B. *Thresholds of the Mind: Your Personal Roadmap to Success, Happiness, and Contentment*. Beaverton: Centerpointe Press, 2007.

Harris, B. The Truth Behind Holosync and Other Neurotechnologies. Retrieved Sept. 22, 2009 from http://www.integralrecovery.com/articles/the-science-behind-holsync-and-other-neurotechnologies.

Hutchison, M. *Mega Brain: New Tools and Techniques for Brain Growth and Mind Expansion*. New York: Ballantine Books, 1991.

Knack, W. A. Psychotherapy and Alcoholics Anonymous: An Integrated Report. *Journal of Psychotherapy Integration*, 1, 86–109. Doi: 10.1037/a0015447, 2009.

McCauley, K. (Audio CD). *The Disease Model of Addiction–Part 1*.

Miller, W. R., and S. Rollnick. *Motivational Interviewing. Preparing People for Change*. New York: The Guilford Press, 2002.

Mellen, R. R., and M. Wade. Reducing Sheriff's Officers' Symptoms of Depression Using Cranial Electrotherapy Stimulation (C.E.S): A Control Experimental Study, 2008. Retrieved September 22, 2009 from http://www.alphastim.com/repository/assets/pdf/mellon_CES2.pdf.

Riso, D. R., and R. Hudson. *The Wisdom of the Enneagram*. New York: Bantam Books, 1999.

Wahbeh, H., C. Calabrese, and H. Zwickey. Binaural beat technology in humans: A pilot study to assess psychological and physiological effects. *Journal of Alternative and Complementary Medicine* 1, 25–32. DOI: 10.1089/acm.2006.6196, 2007.

Wilber, K. *Integral Psychology: Consciousness, Spirit, Psychology, Therapy*. Boston: Shambhala Publishing, 2000.

Appendix 4

Integral Recovery Twelve Steps

1. I acknowledge that I have a problem and that because of _____, my life has become unmanageable.

2. I take full responsibility for this problem and am willing to do the work necessary to heal.

3. I am coming to believe that there is a way out, and that the way out consists of an Integral Recovery Practice that simultaneously exercises my body, mind, heart, and soul.

4. I am ready to conduct a comprehensive evaluation of my past and find the source of my pain, fear, and suffering.

5. Having found the source of this pain, I am willing to release it.

6. Having found and identified the sources of my trauma and suffering, I am willing to do the healing work that is available and necessary for my continued growth and happiness.

7. I made a list of everyone and everything that I have harmed as a result of my unconscious and compulsive behaviors.

8. I made restitution and reconciliation wherever wisely and compassionately possible.

9. As a part of my awakening process, I am examining my core beliefs, my values, and my life callings.

10. I continue to examine my ego structure with rigorous honesty and how my unconscious maps and stories limit or empower my life's progress and unfolding.

11. I continue to evaluate my Integral Recovery Practice and make changes or adjustments as necessary.

12. As a result of this awakening journey, I commit myself to a life of integrity and service

Notes

Introduction

1. Joseph A. Califano, *High Society: How Substance Abuse Ravages America and What to Do About It* (New York: Public Affairs,™ a member of the Perseus Books Group, 2007).

2. Califano, p. xii.

3. http://www.nida.nih.gov/about/welcome/aboutdrugabuse/magnitude.

4. The largest research institute at Brandeis, hosting several national policy centers that focus on health care financing, behavioral health, and international health.

5. These numbers are always in debate, as the percentage varies from study to study.

6. Author, philosopher, and founder of the Integral Institute.

7. See Fritjof Capra's pioneering work *The Tao of Physics* and the many similar volumes that followed in its wake.

8. Passages to Recovery closed its doors in July 2011.

9. "Introduction to Integral Theory and Practice: The AQAL Map," published on the integralnaked.org website.

10. When I say Integral map, I am referring to the AQAL map (pronounced ah-qwul), which is an acronym for all quadrants, all lines, all levels, all states, and all types. Throughout this book, I use the terms "Integral map" and "AQAL map" interchangeably.

11. As Integral scholar Sean Hargens once said, it takes x amount of years to understand Integral, because the more we look the more we see.

12. The Integral, or AQAL, model, so the story goes, originally came about as a response to the overwhelming amount of information Ken Wilber had collected, and was then faced with, as he was writing his opus magnum, *Sex, Ecology, Spirituality: The Spirit of Evolution*. As Wilber relates it, he was dealing with many types of hierarchies—hierarchies of atoms; molecules; cultural hierarchies; spiritual hierarchies; biological and psychological hierarchies, etc. They

were written down on pieces of legal paper pasted all over his walls. Wilber knew they somehow related but couldn't figure out how. Then, presto! One of those vision/logic moments happened (as when I first saw the vision of Integral Recovery), and Wilber saw the four quadrants.

At that moment, Wilber realized how all the different hierarchies that arise in the universe could be organized and how they relate to each other. And that was the beginning of the Integral model. Wilber's genius didn't stop with the four quadrants (I have often thought they would be enough of a contribution for one lifetime). From there, he went on to add lines, stages (levels), states, and types, and if he left anything essential out, I haven't been able to find it. Clearly, Wilber did not invent all the categories included in the Integral model, but, being the great Integralist that he is, he was able to combine all of these elements in such a way as to deepen our understanding of individual parts and how they fit together, causing a revolutionary birth of intellectual enlightenment. So, what we now have is a way of looking at reality, or any part thereof, that is more profound and more complete than any prior approach.

13. Matthew Fox, *The Reinvention of Work: A New Vision of Livelihood for our Time* (San Francisco: HarperSanFrancisco, 1995).

14. This bias toward hiring recovering addicts to help other addicts is due almost completely to the huge influence of AA in the field of recovery. The idea is that only an addict can understand another addict—hence, the AA distrust of therapy and "experts."

15. www.IntegralNaked.org

16. This essay was later expanded into the pocket-sized book *The Integral Vision: A Very Short Introduction to the Revolutionary Integral Approach to Life, God, the Universe, and Everything* (Boston: Shambhala, 2007).

Chapter 1

1. *Alcoholics Anonymous: Big Book* (New York: Alcoholics Anonymous World Services, Inc., 1939).

2. The National Center on Addiction and Substance Abuse at Columbia University (CASA) Press Releases: 2010, *Behind Bars II: Substance Abuse and America's Prison Population*. Lauren Duran and Sulaiman Beg, contacts. CASAColumbia.org: News Room: Press Releases.

3. J. Olds and P. Milner "Positive Reinforcement Produced by Electrical Stimulation of Septal Area and Other Regions of Rat Brain," *Journal of Comparative and Physiological Psychology* 47 (1954): 419–27; J. Olds, "Pleasure Centers in the Brain," *Scientific American* (October, 1956), reprinted in S. Coopersmith, ed., Frontiers of Psychological Research, (San Francisco: Freeman, 1966), 54–59.

4. New research using the latest brain scanning technologies reveals how this hijacking of the dopamine regulation system in the midbrain actually causes

physical changes in the lower neocortex, in which the neocortex sends messages back to the reptilian brain stem, saying that the only thing that should be rewarded by dopamine at this point is more drugs. It has become clear that dopamine is not merely about what is pleasurable, but about what is essential and important. At this point, it is not love, or family, God, country, sports, sex, or anything else that is important. Only the drug. All other behaviors, thoughts, and feelings revolve around the central axis—the drug. This explains the moral, spiritual, and intellectual deterioration of the addict and why drugs become the one and only thing that have meaning and matter anymore. Dr. Nora Volkow, Director of the National Institute on Drug Abuse, is one of the leading scientists in the area of addiction research.

5. Joseph A. Califano, *High Society* (New York: Public Affairs™, a member of the Perseus Books Group, 2007). Source Notes, p. 230. According to OAS, SAMHSA, Results from the 2005 National Survey of Drug Use and Health: National Findings, DHHS Pub. No. SMA 06–4194 (Rockville, MD): DHHS, SAMHSA, OAS, 2006.

6. Califano, *High Society*.

7. A wonderful cinemagraphic example of this is the very powerful film *Train Spotting*, which I highly recommend.

8. When the National Institute on Drug Abuse reviewed the body of "outcome studies" comparing court-mandated to voluntary patients, they found no measurable statistical difference in success rates, even though coerced patients stayed in treatment longer. Maia Szalavitz writing in *City Limits Weekly*, July/ August 2001 is a co-author of *Recovery Options: The Complete Guide: How You and Your Loved Ones Can Understand and Treat Alcohol and Other Drug Problems* (Wiley, 2000).

9. The other side of the coin, studied by Miller and C'de Baca (1994), describes sudden personality change occurring in a positive sense—an Ebenezer Scrooge-like transformation. I have often seen this with my students, when, in short order, I would see an extraordinarily fine human being resurface from the addictive trance. In both cases, the change happens rapidly, is dramatic, and is absolutely noticeable to those in relationship with the transforming individual. See William R. Miller and Janet C'de Baca, *Quantum Change: When Epiphanies and Sudden Insights Transform Ordinary Lives* (New York: Guilford, 2001).

10. This could be either conscious stress or unconscious stress, as in a repressed traumatic memory.

11. Cortisol and hormones such as adrenaline increase blood pressure, and some studies suggest that in cases of severe stress, the effects go beyond increasing blood pressure to actually injure the cells of the body and their ability to heal, accelerating the aging process.

12. Dawson Church, *The Genie in Your Genes: Epigenetic Medicine and the New Biology of Intention*. (Santa Rosa, CA: Elite Books, 2007), p. 37.

13. See appendix I from Califano, *High Society*, p. 187.

14. Dr. Hans Selye, pioneering scientist on the nature of stress, authored *The Stress of Life* and *Stress without Distress* in the 1970s and submitted his manuscript, "The Nature of Stress" to a colleague before he died in 1982. Selye's famous and revolutionary concept of stress opened countless avenues of treatment through the discovery that hormones participate in the development of many degenerative diseases.

15. I've adapted items 1 through 4 from Chris Prentiss, *The Alcoholism Addiction Cure* (California: Power, 2005). Prentiss offers an impressive and effective approach to treating addiction, for which I have great respect. In my opinion, he only lacks the clarity and comprehensive structure that an AQAL framework, combined with an Integral Recovery Practice, provides. I have added items 5 and 6 based on personal experience.

16. With binaural brainwave entrainment technology, we can entrain our brain waves to the desired brainwave state—in our case, a deeply meditative state—simply by listening, with headphones, to an audio track, which plays a different beat into each ear. I will discuss this technology at length in future chapters.

17. There is an ever-growing body of literature on the subject of trauma and addiction. It is impossible to include all of the references; however, the following are a representative sample of this large body of associative literature:

Addictions and Trauma Recovery: Healing the Body, Mind and Spirit. Miller, Dusty; Guidry, Laurie. New York, New York, U.S.: Norton, 2001. *Trauma and Addiction Experiences of African American Women.* Ruth E. Davis, Millersville University, Millersville, PA.; Judy E. Mill-R.N.; Janice M. Roper-R.N.-Ph.D., West Los Angeles VA Medical Center, Los Angeles, CA. *Western Journal of Nursing Research,* August 1997, Volume 19, No. 4, pages 442–465. *An Exploratory Study of Rape Survivors' Prescription Drug Use as a Means of Coping with Sexual Assault.* Marisa L. Sturza, Rebecca Campbell, Dept. of Psychology, Michigan State University. Psychology of Women Quarterly, Dec. 1, 2005, Volume 21, No. 4, pages 353–63.

18. Viktor E. Frankl, *Man's Search for Meaning* (New York: Simon and Schuster, 1959; first published in Austria in 1946 under the title *Ein Psycholog erlebt das Konzentrationslager*).

19. William Glasser, M.D., *Choice Theory: A New Psychology of Personal Freedom* (New York: HarperCollins, 1998).

Chapter 2

1. Image courtesy of Integral Institute.

2. Founded in 1996 by veteran management consultant, trainer, and best-selling author David Allen (*Getting Things Done: The Art of Stress-Free Productiv-*

ity), the company provides seminars, coaching, and products that facilitate the implementation of the best practices of productive work. See the David Allen Company at www.davidco.com.

Chapter 3

1. Image courtesy of Integral Institute.

2. Dr. Susanne Cook-Greuter, born in Switzerland, is the principal of the consulting firm Cook-Greuter and Associates. She holds a doctorate in education from Harvard University and is an internationally known authority on mature adult development. Her thesis, *Postautonomous Ego Development* (1999), is a landmark study in the characteristics and assessment of highly developed and influential individuals and leaders. Dr. Cook-Greuter is also a founding member of Ken Wilber's Integral Institute. In addition to publishing many papers, she has coauthored two books on adult development, creativity, and spirituality: *Creativity, Spirituality, and Transcendence: Paths to Integrity and Wisdom in the Mature Self* (1999), and *Transcendence and Mature Thought in Adulthood* (1994).

3. *Sex, Ecology, Spirituality*, p. 263.

4. See Don Beck and Christopher Cowan, *Spiral Dynamics: Mastering Values, Leadership, and Change* (Malden, MA: Blackwell, 1996).

5. In Integral theory, we use many different developmental models. In Integral Recovery, however, I have chosen Spiral Dynamics as our developmental entry point for its beautiful applicability to the journey of recovery and its ability to help us understand not only individual development but also our development as a species, as well as the many often conflicting moral perspectives that abound in our world. There are, however, many other developmental models, such as those developed by Susanne Cook-Greuter and Robert Kegan, that are perhaps more empirical in their research basis. But I have found that Spiral Dynamics is an exceptional introductory model and finds immediate resonance with my students, addicts, adolescents, and their families.

Keep in mind that Spiral Dynamics is measuring only one line: that of values. In conversation with Ken Wilber, Wilber agreed that Spiral Dynamics is an excellent place to start when it comes to developmental stages, but is by no means the end of the story. Wilber, in his brilliant and highly recommended work, *Integral Psychology*, places in the appendix of the book over a hundred different developmental models ranging from premodern to modern to postmodern. Here we see that there is a commonality among all of these developmental models in that the projection of growth always tends to move from simple to more complex as we move up the developmental ladder, with each senior level having the capacity to transcend but at the same time include the levels of development that preceded it.

6. Image courtesy of Steve Self (www.formlessmountain.com).

7. It should be noted that Ken Wilber later developed a stage model using a different color system than Beck. Wilber's color system follows the spectrum of the rainbow and in some places still corresponds with Beck's model. For example, orange is still orange, and green is still green. There are some subtle differences between Wilber's and Beck's model, chief among which is Wilber's presentation of a third tier of development.

8. See the Homeric literary masterpieces the *Illiad* and the *Odyssey*, paying special attention to the characters of Achilles and Agamemnon.

9. As Sgt. Friday from the sixties television series *Dragnet* used to say.

10. Recently, I heard an Episcopalian priest, Cynthia Bourgeault, say that the Vatican II and the Beatles were the harbingers of the Green emergence.

11. Robert Kegan, *The Evolving Self: Problem and Process in Human Development* (Cambridge, MA: Harvard University Press, 1982).

12. There is a part of us, or perhaps a force in us, which some identify as Eros, that longs for and strives for health and higher evolutionary growth. But, in most cases, and especially in the case of addicts, I believe it is divine discontent that creates the channels through which this evolutionary Eros can flow.

13. Christina Hoff Sommers, *The War against Boys* (New York: Simon and Schuster, 2000).

14. As Napoleon is quoted, "A solider will fight long and hard for a bit of colored ribbon." Or again, "Give me enough medals and I will win every war." (Napoleon knew his Red soldiers.)

15. Ilya Prigogine and Isabelle Stengers, *Order out of Chaos: Man's New Dialogue with Nature* (New York: Bantam, 1984).

16. The statistics noted in the following sections are from Dr. Don Beck's dialogue on integralnaked.org. See also Beck's website Spiral Dynamics Integral at www.spiraldynamics.net.

Chapter 4

1. Howard Gardner, *Frames of Mind: The Theory of Multiple Intelligences* (New York: Basic Books, 1993).

2. Normally, in Integral circles we speak of the four essential self-related lines: body, mind, emotional/shadow, and spiritual. But for our purposes in Integral Recovery, I have added a fifth, the ethical line, because the disease of addiction so negatively affects the addict's moral and ethical sense.

3. Cindy Wigglesworth has developed a Spiritual Intelligence (SQ) test; see her website www.consciouspursuits.com. And you will find links to test Emotional Intelligence (EQ) at www.integralstrategies.org/tests.html. See also Ken Wilber's Integral Operating System DVD, accessible at www.integrallife.com, in which he

discusses psychographs, how most of us are uneven in our line development, and how this can be corrected by Integral practice.

4. George Leonard and Michael Murphy, *The Life We Are Given: A Long-term Program for Realizing the Potential of Body, Mind, Heart, and Soul* (New York: Tarcher/Putnam, 1995).

5. Ken Wilber, *The Integral Vision: A Very Short Introduction to the Revolutionary Integral Approach to Life, God, the Universe, and Everything* (Boston: Shambhala, 2007).

6. A practicing psychiatrist born in 1925, Glasser has authored and coauthored numerous books on mental health, one of the most influential of which was his early work *Reality Therapy: A New Approach to Psychiatry*, published by Colophon Books in 1975.

7. Daniel J. Siegel, M.D., *Mindsight: The New Science of Transformation* (New York: Random House, 2010).

8. This is meditation with the aid of brainwave entrainment technology, the benefits of which I will describe in detail in future chapters.

9. In Wilber speak, an injunction is an actual practice—something you do in order to learn or understand something, such as practicing meditation to understand your interiors and essence or looking through a telescope to gain a greater understanding of the universe.

10. The Profound Meditation Program, brainwave entrainment technology, and contemplative and meditation techniques, to include work on the shadow.

11. Viktor E. Frankl, *Man's Search for Meaning* (New York: Simon and Schuster, 1959; first published in Austria in 1946 under the title *Ein Psycholog erlebt das Konzentrationslager*).

12. Logotherapy (derived from the Greek word, "logos," which is defined as "meaning") is considered the "Third Viennese School of Psychotherapy."

13. I am a masculine-identified Six on the Enneagram, which means I have a highly developed sense of mission and responsibility. For others, the fallback position of looking and feeling good may indeed help!

14. Since beginning my healing journey with binaural brainwave entrainment technology, I have tested and used many of the binaural products available. In 2010, I met Eric Thompson, a brilliant pioneer and innovator in this field. We went on to form our own company, iAwake Technologies, and began to produce our own audio transformative products. These include BWE along with other audio technologies. Our commitment is to keep evolving this technology and to make it better and affordable to the many, as well as providing support and education for those using the technology. iAwake's flagship product is the Profound Meditation Program. Since our inception in 2010, we have received extraordinarily positive and exciting reports and accounts from all over the world from those who have been using this technology. See www.profoundmeditationprogram.com for more information.

15. Published on the Integral Recovery website, the Integral Life website, and the Integrales Forum website (Spirituelle Lehrer: Millsteine, Verantwortung und Liebe).

Chapter 5

1. Ken Wilber, *The Integral Operating System*:Version 1.0. CDs, DVD, workbook. Boulder: Sounds True, 2005.

2. Binaural brainwave entrainment is accomplished using a simple stereo headset and CD player; one beat is played into the left ear, and a different beat is played into the right ear. The brain wants to make sense of the discrepancy in the two beats, say 100 and 110 beats per minute, so it splits the difference to a "phantom" beat of, say, 5 hertz. This entrains your brain waves at the very low brainwave state of 5 hertz, in this case, to which the corresponding brainwave state is theta, the state associated with REM/dream sleep.

3. Bill Harris, *Thresholds of the Mind* (Beaverton, OR: Centerpointe Press, 2002). The various producers of binaural brainwave entrainment technology all seem to have come to this conclusion.

4. Author of *The Way of the Superior Man* (Boulder: Sounds True, Inc., 1997, 2004).

5. The word endogenous derives from the Greek: ενδογενής, meaning "proceeding from within" ("ενδο"=inside "-γενής"=coming from), the complement of exogenous (Greek: εξωγενής exo, "έξω"= outside) "proceeding from outside."

6. Psychiatrist, philosopher, and author of *Essential Spirituality: The 7 Central Practices to Awaken Heart and Mind.*

7. The Sedona Method is a method that trains one in how to do emotional releasing work. See Hale Dwoskin's book, *The Sedona Method* (Sedona, AZ: Sedona, 2003).

8. Sevens on the Enneagram are referred to as the epicures or hedonists. In their unhealthy aspect, there can be a pathological avoidance of anything that is painful or uncomfortable.

9. Robert Lyons.

Chapter 6

1. Charlotte Davis Kasl, *Many Roads, One Journey: Moving beyond the 12 Steps* (New York: HarperCollins, 1992).

2. David Deida's work is exemplary in this area. See David Deida, *The Way of the Superior Man* (Boulder: Sounds True, 2005).

3. Here I have used the type descriptions presented in the excellent *The Enneagram for the Spirit: How to Make Peace with Your Personality and Understand Others* by Mary Horsley, published by Barron's Educational Series in 2005. See Horsley's website at www.maryhorsley.co.uk.

4. Excellent books on the Enneagram include *The Wisdom of the Enneagram* by Riso and Hudson; *The Enneagram Made Easy* by Baron and Wagele; *Personality Types* by Riso and Hudson; *The Enneagram: Understanding Yourself and the Others in Your Life* by Helen Palmer; *The Enneagram in Love and Work: Understanding Your Intimate and Business Relationships* by Helen Palmer; and *Facets of Unity: The Enneagram of Holy Ideas* by A. H. Almaas.

Chapter 7

1. Motivational interviewing is a directive, client-centered counseling style for eliciting behavior change by helping clients to explore and resolve ambivalence. See William R. Miller and Stephen Rollnick, *Motivational Interviewing* (New York: Guilford, 2002).

2. The existing data on using binaural brainwave entrainment and similar technologies for the treatment of addiction is very encouraging. The first thing I read on this that really excited me was in Michael Hutchison's book *Mega Brain Power*, chapter 26, which was based on the work of William Beckwith, Ph.D., clinical neuropsychologist, and others. Over the past six years, as I have become known for using this type of technology for the treatment of addiction and depression, I have received large amounts of anecdotal data that are extraordinarily positive.

Since I became CEO of iAwake Technologies in 2010, with the worldwide sales of the Profound Meditation Program, I receive almost daily accounts of what is occurring in peoples' lives as they use this technology for various complaints and disorders, including addiction, depression, and ADHD, attesting to its positive transformative powers.

See also Michael M. Hutchison, *Mega Brain: New Tools and Techniques for Brain Growth and Mind Expansion* (New York: Morrow, 1986); and Bill Harris, "The Science Behind Holosync® and Other Neurotechnologies" (Beaverton, OR: Centerpointe Research Institute, 2009).

3. H. Wahbeh, C. Calabrese, H. Zwickey, "Binaural Beat Technology in Humans: A Pilot Study to Assess Psychological and Physiologic Effects," *Journal of Alternative and Complementary Medicine* 13, no. 1 (2007): 25–32; H. Wahbeh, C. Calabrese, H. Zwickey, J. Zajdel "Binaural Beat Technology in Humans: A Pilot Study to Assess Neuropsychologic, Physiologic, And Electroencephalographic Effects," *Journal of Alternative and Complementary Medicine* 13, no. 2 (2007): 199–206: G. Oster, "Auditory beats in the brain" *Sci. Am.* 229, no. 4 (1973):

94–102; D. Fitzpatrick et al.,"Processing Temporal Modulations in Binaural and Monaural Auditory Stimuli by Neurons in the Inferior Colliculus and Auditory Cortex," *JARO* 10, no. 4 (2009): 579–93.

4. The National Center on Addiction and Substance Abuse at Columbia University, *Women under the Influence* (Johns Hopkins University Press, 2006).

5. Daniel J. Siegel, M.D. *Mindsight: The New Science of Transformation* (New York: Random House, 2010).

6. Recorded affirmations are recorded phrases that one listens to as a type of meditation, which describe ideas and images that one would like to instill more deeply into the conscious and unconscious mind in order to promote healing and optimal performance.

7. Leonard, George, and Michael Murphy, *The Life We Are Given: A Long-term Program for Realizing the Potential of Body, Mind, Heart, and Soul* (New York: Jeremy P. Tarcher/Putnam, 1995).

8. K. C. Russell, *The Therapeutic Alliance*. Summary of research in the Outdoor Behavioral Healthcare Research Cooperative from 1999–2006. Technical Report 2, February 2007, Outdoor Behavioral Healthcare Research Cooperative, College of Education and Human Development, University of Minnesota, Minneapolis, MN. 52 pp.

9. Roshi Baker, born Richard Baker, is an American Soto Zen master, Dharma heir to Shunryu Suzuki.

10. William R. Miller and Stephen Rollnick, *Motivational Interviewing* (New York: Guilford, 2002).

Chapter 8

1. Shawn Phillips, *Strength for Life* (New York: Ballantine Books, 2008).

2. Bill Phillips, *Body for Life* (New York: HarperCollins, 1999).

3. Y. Kaufman, et al., "Cognitive Decline in Alzheimer Disease: Impact of Spirituality, Religiosity, and QOL." *Neurology* 68 (2007): 1509–14; N. Lautenschlager et al. (2008) "Effect of Physical Activity on Cognitive Function in Older Adults at Risk for Alzheimer's Disease," *Journal of the American Medical Association* 300, no. 9 (2008): 1027–37; M. P. Mattson et al. "Prophylactic Activation of Neuroprotective Stress Response Pathways by Dietary and Behavioral Manipulations," *NeuroRx* 1 (2004): 112; J. Weuve et al., "Physical Activity, Including Walking, and Cognitive Function in Older Women." *Journal of the American Medical Association* 292, no. 12 (2004): 1454–61; A. V. Witte, "Caloric Restriction Improves Memory in Elderly Humans," *Proceedings of the National Academy of Science*, 106, no. 4(2009): 1255–60; K. Yurko-Mauro, "Results of the MIDAS Trial: Effects of Docosahexaenoic Acid on Physiological and Safety Parameters in Age-Related Cognitive Decline." *Alzheimer's and Dementia* 4 (2009): 84.

4. The brand that I use, Alive! is made by Nature's Way.

5. Sun seems to be a good brand.

6. Made by the company Now.

7. Thomas J. Slaga and Robin Keuneke, *The Detox Revolution* (New York: McGraw-Hill Books, 2003), 47.

8. See Shawn Phillips' "Full Strength" shake in *Strength for Life.*

9. Ken Wilber, Terry Patton, Adam Leonard, and Marco Morelli, *Integral Life Practice: A 21st-Century Blueprint for Physical Health, Emotional Balance, Mental Clarity, and Spiritual Awakening* (Boston: Integral Books, an imprint of Shambhala, 2008).

Chapter 9

1. Bill Harris, *Thresholds of the Mind* (Beaverton, OR: Centerpointe Research Institute, 2007).

2. E. G. Peniston and P. J. Kulkowski, "Alpha-Theta Brainwave Training and Beta-endorphin Levels in Alcoholics," *Alcoholism* 13 (1989): 271–79.

3. E. G. Peniston and P. J. Kulkowski, "Alpha-Theta Brainwave Training and Beta-endorphin Levels in Alcoholics," *Alcoholism* 13 (1989): 271–79.

4. As I mentioned in chapter 1, Dr. Hans Selye, pioneering scientist on the nature of stress, authored *The Stress of Life* and *Stress without Distress* in the 1970s and submitted his manuscript, *The Nature of Stress* to a colleague before he died in 1982. Selye's famous and revolutionary concept of stress opened countless avenues of treatment through the discovery that hormones participate in the development of many degenerative diseases.

5. If you go to the website, www.profoundmeditationprogram.com, you can experience a free demo of this technology and begin your own transformational journey.

6. Daniel L. Kirsch and Marshall Gilula, *Cranial Electrotherapy Stimulation in the Treatment of Depression—Part 1: Practical Pain Management* 7, no. 4 (2007):33–41; *Part 2:* 7, no. 5 (2007): 32–40.

7. A panel of distinguished doctors is currently the Medical Advisory Board for Fisher Wallace Laboratories, producers of the Stimulator. See the Fisher Wallace website for details (www.fisherwallace.com).

8. Daniel L. Kirsch and Marshall Gilula *Cranial Electrotherapy Stimulation in the Treatment of Depression—Part 1: Practical Pain Management* 7, no. 4 (2007):33–41. *Part 2:* 7, no. 5 (2007): 32–40.

9. See also Ray B. Smith, Ph.D., *Cranial Electrotherapy Stimulation: Its First Fifty Years, Plus Three: A Monograph* (Mustang, Oklahoma: Tate, 2007).

10. In 1942, Conrad Waddington coined the term "epigenetics" for "the branch of biology which studies the causal interactions between genes and their

products which bring the phenotype into being" (C. H. Waddington (1942) (1977) *The Epigenotype: Endeavor 1*, 18–20). Today many researchers would define it as inherited changes in phenotype without DNA sequence change.

11. Dawson Church, Ph.D., *The Genie in Your Genes: Epigenetic Medicine and the New Biology of Intention* (Santa Rosa, CA: Elite Books, 2007), p. 37.

12. A mirror neuron is a neuron that fires both when an animal acts and when the animal observes the same action performed by another. Thus, the neuron "mirrors" the behavior of the other, as though the observer were itself acting. See Giacomo Rizzolatti and Laila Craighero, "The Mirror-Neuron System," *Annual Review of Neuroscience* 27 (2004): 169–92. Christian Keysers, *The Empathic Brain: How the Discovery of Mirror Neurons Changes Our Understanding of Human Nature,* Kindle Edition, 2011. V. S. Ramachandran, "Mirror Neurons and Imitation Learning as the Driving Force behind 'the Great Leap Forward' in Human Evolution." Edge Foundation. Retrieved 2006.

13. Dawson Church, Ph.D. *The Genie in Your Genes: Epigenetic Medicine and the New Biology of Intention* (Santa Rosa, CA: Elite Books, 2007).

14. I will examine Leonard's types of practitioners in detail in chapter 12, "Practice and the Path to Mastery."

15. The superego is the part of the human psyche that tells us what we *should* do, according to Freud.

Chapter 10

1. The 3-2-1 Shadow Process is explained in depth in the Integral Life Practice Starter Kit. See also http://integrallife.com/video/3-2-1-shadow-process.

2. Hale Dwoskin, *The Sedona Method* (Sedona: Sedona Press, 2003).

3. Elisha Goldstein, Ph.D. *Mindful Solutions* audio CD. Elisha Goldstein is a psychologist and teacher of Mindfulness-Based Stress Reduction in the San Francisco Bay Area. See www.drsgoldstein.com.

4. For a synopsis of Jung's main concepts, including the Shadow archetype, see the Institute of Transpersonal Psychology website, www.itp.edu/about/carl_jung.php.

5. Hale Dwoskin, *The Sedona Method* (Sedona: Sedona Press, 2003).

6. From the beginning of Kelly Sosan Bearer's excellent instructions on how to do the 3-2-1 Shadow Process on the Integral Chicks website, http://www.integralchicks.com/2010/06/the-3-2-1-shadow-process/.

7. Sean Esbjörn-Hargens is an Integral theorist associated with Ken Wilber and a founding member of Integral Institute.

8. *The Essential Rumi*, translated by Coleman Barks (Castle Books, 1995).

9. Arjuna Ardagh, *The Translucent Revolution: How People Just Like You Are Waking Up and Changing the World* (Novato, CA: New World Library, 2005). This

book is highly recommended to anyone interested in a deeper understanding of Integral Recovery.

Chapter 11

1. Ken Wilber explores this idea in great detail in his book, *The Marriage of Sense and Soul: Integrating Science and Religion*. Here, he deconstructs the popular idea of a paradigm as an intellectual structure that we come up with to reinvent our reality and see things differently. Ken clearly shows how this is a new age fallacy and misinterpretation of Thomas Kuhn's seminal work about paradigms, *The Structure of Scientific Revolutions*. Wilber and Kuhn both show how paradigm shifts come, not from mere new theoretical frameworks, but from actual injunctions. For example, when the telescope was invented, it gave us a new window into the nature of the universe. The injunction was to look through the telescope into the heavens and collect the data provided by the new technology. This, in turn, absolutely shattered the old paradigms and gave rise to a completely new paradigm in which the earth was no longer the center of the universe, merely a small part of a much larger system. Another example would be the invention of the microscope and the ensuing realization that there exists an entire world of previously unknown life forms, which coexist with us and are hugely determinant in our lives as human beings.

2. Maslow's hierarchy of needs is a theory in psychology, proposed by Abraham Maslow in *A Theory of Human Motivation* (1943).

3. http://psychology.about.com/od/theoriesofpersonality/a/hierarchyneeds.htm.

4. Albert Schweitzer (January 14, 1875–September 4, 1965), philosopher, physician, and humanitarian.

5. William Hutchinson Murray (1913–1996), from his 1951 book entitled *The Scottish Himalayan Expedition*. (This quote is often mistakenly attributed to Goethe.)

6. The Oxford Group was a Christian movement that had a following in Europe and America in the 1920s and 1930s. Both Bill Wilson and Bob Smith, the two founders of AA, were members of the Oxford Group.

7. Arjuna Ardagh, *The Translucent Revolution: How People Just Like You Are Waking Up and Changing the World* (Novato, CA: New World Library, 2005).

8. Karen Armstrong, *A History of God* (New York: Random House, 1993).

9. Published by Integral Books, an imprint of Shambhala, 2006.

10. There is no historical evidence that St. Francis ever wrote the prayer, but whatever the source, it seems to have nailed the spirit and essence of the man, who is one of my all-time spiritual heroes.

11. The Prayer of St. Francis is a Christian prayer attributed to the thirteenth-century Saint Francis of Assisi.

Chapter 12

1. Daniel Coyle, *The Talent Code: Greatness Isn't Born. It's Grown. Here's How* (New York: Random House, 2009); Geoff Colvin, *Talent Is Overrated: What Really Separates World-Class Performers from Everybody Else* (New York: Penguin Group, 2008); Marilyn Mandala Schlitz, Cassandra Vieten, and Tina Amorok, *Living Deeply: The Art and Science of Transformation in Everyday Life* (Oakland: New Harbinger Publications and Noetic Books, 2007); David Shenk, *The Genius in All of Us: New Insights into Genetics, Talent, and IQ* (New York: Random House, 2009).

2. Geoff Colvin, *Talent Is Overrated: What Really Separates World-Class Performers from Everybody Else* (New York: Penguin Group, 2008), chs. 2, 4.

3. David Shenk, *The Genius in All of Us: New Insights into Genetics, Talent, and IQ* (New York: Random House, 2009).

4. The Nobel Prize in Literature in 1953 was awarded to Winston Churchill "for his mastery of historical and biographical description as well as brilliant oratory in defending exalted human values."

5. The Royal Military Academy Sandhurst is, however, a two-year college as opposed to the four-year West Point.

6. From David Shenk's *The Genius in All of Us.*

7. For more on this subject, see Ken Wilber's *The Marriage of Sense and Soul: Integrating Science and Religion.*

8. Aldous Huxley, *The Perennial Philosophy* (New York: HarperCollins, 1944).

9. George Leonard, *Mastery: The Keys to Success and Long-Term Fulfillment* (New York: Penguin Books, 1992).

10. George Leonard and Michael Murphy, *The Life We Are Given: A Long-term Program for Realizing the Potential of Body, Mind, Heart, and Soul* (New York: Tarcher/Putnam, 1995).

11. Ben Hogan, generally considered one of the greatest golfers in the history of the game, went professional in 1930.

12. Ken Wilber, *The Eye of Spirit: An Integral Vision for a World Gone Slightly Mad* (Boston: Shambhala, 2001, 2000), p. 65.

13. E. G. Peniston and P. J. Kulkowski, "Alpha-Theta Brainwave Training and Beta-endorphin Levels in Alcoholics," *Alcoholism* 13 (1989): 271–79.

14. Brian Thomas Swimme is on the faculty of the California Institute of Integral Studies, in San Francisco, where he teaches evolutionary cosmology to graduate students in the humanities. Swimme brings the context of story to our understanding of the 13.7-billion-year trajectory of cosmogenesis. His published work includes *The Universe Is a Green Dragon* (Bear and Company, 1984), *The Universe Story* (Harper San Francisco, 1992), written with Thomas Berry, and *The Hidden Heart of the Cosmos* (Orbis, 1996). Swimme is the producer of three DVD series: *Canticle to the Cosmos, The Earth's Imagination,* and *The Powers of the Universe.*

15. George Leonard, *Mastery: The Keys to Success and Long-Term Fulfillment* (New York: Penguin Books, 1992).

16. *Living Deeply*, p. 209.

17. Sir Winston Churchill (1874–1965).

Chapter 14

1. Willow Pearson, Integral teacher and musician.

2. In the near future, I plan to design and release an Integral Recovery Relapse Prevention Tool Kit app.

Appendix 1

1. See Ken Wilber, Foreword to *Integral Medicine: A Noetic Reader*, at http://www.kenwilber.com/writings/index?category=Forewords.

2. Ken Wilber, *The Integral Vision* (Boston: Shambhala, 2007).

3. Ken Wilber, *Integral Psychology* (Boston: Shambhala, 2000).

4. Ken Wilber, *Sex, Ecology, Spirituality: The Spirit of Evolution* (Boston: Shambhala, 1995).

5. I especially recommend the works of Riso and Hudson and Helen Palmer. I also highly recommend the services of Leslie Hershberger, M.A., who is extraordinarily gifted at helping people find and understand their types. Hershberger has taught Integral Recovery students online via Skype, awakening students to their unconscious and habitual patterns of behavior and relating, for which my students have always been very grateful.

6. A practicing psychiatrist, he has also authored and coauthored numerous influential books on mental health, counseling, and the improvement of schools and teaching and several publications advocating a public health approach to mental health versus the prevailing "medical" model.

Appendix 2

1. Some approaches to dealing with alcoholism are Rational Recovery, Smart Recovery, Women in Sobriety, and of course all of the 12-step–based groups.

2. In a very recent conversation with a third-year medical student, while doing the final edits on this book, I asked what she had learned about the disease of addiction, and she replied that there definitely seemed to be a genetic component and that it is a neurological disorder. So, as one of my favorite poets, Bob Dylan, has written, perhaps the times they are a-changin'.

3. Students have told me of their experiences "doctor-shopping," getting Vicodin and Oxycontin for one body part and then more Oxycontin for another body part, and so on. Never underestimate the cunning of addicts when it comes to obtaining these desired substances. Although it is hard to tell the exact percentage of pharmaceuticals that make up the illegal drug trade in the United States, students tell me that it is as high as 50 percent. In other words, 50 percent of illegal drugs now consumed in the United States are pharmaceuticals, both the narcotic pain-killing variety and the "Benzos," such as Valium and Xanax.

4. The first four horsemen are conquest, war, famine, and death, as told in eight verses of the book of Revelation, which is the last book in the Bible. The four horsemen appear when the Lamb (Jesus) opens the first four seals of a scroll with seven seals. As each of the first four seals is opened, a different colored horse and its rider are seen by the apostle John, as described in Revelation 6:1–8.

Appendix 3

1. This appendix originally appeared in the *Journal of Integral Theory and Practice* in a slightly modified form. Coauthor John Dupuy, M.A., is the founder of Integral Recovery. He received his B.A. from Texas State University in modern languages and received his master's degree in transpersonal psychology from John F. Kennedy University. John is the author of numerous articles on Integral Recovery, Integral practice, and spirituality. His articles have been published in the *Journal of Integral Theory and Practice*, on the Integral Life website, and translated into German and published in *Integral Forum* and *Integral Perspectives*. Coauthor Adam Gorman has been in recovery for more than nine years. Adam has worked for numerous wilderness therapy companies, including Open Sky Wilderness Therapy and Passages to Recovery. He received his undergraduate degree in psychology from the Catholic University of America. Adam is currently getting his doctorate in clinical psychology while concurrently earning his master's degree in Integral Theory at John F. Kennedy University. He is presently writing his doctoral dissertation on Integral Recovery and its application in a treatment setting.

2. The following is a firsthand account of the treatment methods used while Esau was under care.

References

Alcoholics Anonymous. *Big Book*. New York: Alcoholics Anonymous World Services, 1939.

Allen, David. *Getting Things Done: The Art of Stress-Free Productivity*. New York: Penguin, 2001.

Almaas, A. H. *Facets of Unity: The Enneagram of Holy Ideas*. Berkeley: Diamond Books, 1998.

Ardagh, Arjuna. *The Translucent Revolution: How People Just Like You Are Waking Up and Changing the World*. Novato, CA: New World Library, 2005.

Barks, Coleman, trans., with John Moyne. *The Essential Rumi*. HarperOne, 1995.

Baron, Renee, and Elizabeth Wagele. *The Enneagram Made Easy: Discover the 9 Types of People*. New York: HarperCollins, 1994.

Beasley, Joseph D., M.D. *Food for Recovery*. New York: Crown, 1994.

Beattie, Melody. *Codependent No More: How to Stop Controlling Others and Start Caring for Yourself*. Center City, MN: Hazelden Foundation, 1986, 1992.

Beck, Don, and Christopher Cowan. *Spiral Dynamics: Mastering Values, Leadership, and Change*. Malden, MA: Blackwell, 1996.

Califano, Joseph A., *High Society: How Substance Abuse Ravages America and What to Do about It*. New York: Public Affairs,™ a member of the Perseus Books Group, 2007.

Campbell, Joseph. *The Hero's Journey*. Novato, CA: New World Library, 1990, 2003.

Capra, Fritjof. *The Tao of Physics: An Exploration of the Parallels between Modern Physics and Eastern Mysticism*. Boston: Shambhala, 1975, 1983, 1991, 1999.

Church, Dawson, Ph.D. *The Genie in Your Genes: Epigenetic Medicine and the New Biology of Intention*. Santa Rosa, CA: Elite Books, 2007.

Clapton, Eric. *Clapton: The Autobiography*. New York: Random House, 2007.

Colvin, Geoff. *Talent Is Overrated: What Really Separates World-Class Performers from Everybody Else*. New York: Penguin Group (USA), 2008.

Cook-Greuter, Susanne, ed. "Postautonomous Ego Development: Its Nature and Measurement" (1999). Doctoral dissertation, Harvard University, 1999. Dissertation Abstracts International, 60 (06), 2000.

Cousens, Gabriel, M.D. *Depression-Free for Life*. New York: HarperCollins, 2000.

Coyle, Daniel, *The Talent Code: Greatness Isn't Born. It's Grown. Here's How*. New York: Random House, 2009.

Cushnir, Howard. *Unconditional Bliss: Finding Happiness in the Face of Hardship*. Wheaton, IL: Theosophical, 2000.

D'Adamo, Peter J., Dr. *Eat Right 4 Your Type*. New York: Putnam's Sons, 1996.

Davis, Ruth E., Judy E. Mill, R.N., Janice M. Roper, R.N. Ph.D. "Trauma and Addiction Experiences of African American Women." West Los Angeles VA Medical Center, Los Angeles, CA. *Western Journal of Nursing Research* 19, no. 4 (August 1997): 442–465.

Deida, David. *The Way of the Superior Man*. Boulder: Sounds True, 1997, 2004.

Dupuy, J., and A. Gorman. "Integral Recovery®: An AQAL Approach to Inpatient Alcohol and Drug Treatment." *Journal of Integral Theory and Practice* 5, no. 3 (2010): 86–101.

Dwoskin, Hale. *The Sedona Method*. Sedona: Sedona, 2003.

Fitzpatrick, D., et al. "Processing Temporal Modulations in Binaural and Monaural Auditory Stimuli by Neurons in the Inferior Colliculus and Auditory Cortex," *JARO* 10, no. 4 (2009): 579–593.

Fox, Matthew. *Creativity: Where the Divine and the Human Meet*. New York: Tarcher/Putnam, 2002.

———. *The Reinvention of Work: A New Vision of Livelihood for our Time*. San Francisco: HarperSanFrancisco, 1995.

Frankl, Viktor E. *Man's Search for Meaning*. New York: Simon and Schuster, 1959.

Gardner, Howard. *Frames of Mind: The Theory of Multiple Intelligences*. New York: Basic Books, 1993.

Glasser, William, M.D. *Choice Theory: A New Psychology of Personal Freedom*. New York: HarperCollins, 1998.

———. *Reality Therapy: A New Approach to Psychiatry*. New York: Harper and Row, 1965, 1975.

Goldstein, Elisha, Ph.D. *Mindful Solutions for Stress, Anxiety, and Depression*. Audio CD, Mindful Solution Series, 2007.

Gregson, David, Jay S. Efran, and G. Alan Marlatt. *The Tao of Sobriety: Helping You to Recover from Alcohol and Drug Addiction*. New York: St. Martin's, 2002.

Guidry, Laurie, and Dusty Miller. *Addictions and Trauma Recovery: Healing the Body, Mind and Spirit*. New York: Norton, 2001.

Harris, Bill. "The Science behind Holosync® and Other Neurotechnologies." Beaverton, OR: Centerpointe Research Institute, 2009.

———. *Thresholds of the Mind: Your Personal Roadmap to Success, Happiness, and Contentment*. Beaverton, OR: Centerpointe Press, 2002.

Homer. *The Iliad*. New York: Penguin, 1950, 2003.

———. *The Odyssey*. New York: Penguin, 1946, 1991.

Horsley, Mary. *The Enneagram for the Spirit: How to Make Peace with Your Personality and Understand Others.* Hauppage, NY: Barron's Educational Series, 2005.

Hutchison, Michael. *Mega Brain Power: Transform Your Life with Mind Machines and Brain Nutrients.* New York: Hyperion Books, 1994.

Huxley, Aldous. *The Perennial Philosophy.* New York: HarperCollins, 1944.

James, William. *The Varieties of Religious Experiences.* New York: Random House, 1994.

Jenkins, Roy. *Churchill: A Biography.* New York: Farrar, Straus and Giroux, 2001.

Kasl, Charlotte Davis. *Many Roads, One Journey: Moving Beyond the 12 Steps.* New York: HarperCollins, 1992.

Kegan, Robert. *The Evolving Self: Problem and Process in Human Development.* Cambridge, MA: Harvard University Press, 1982.

————, and Lisa L. Lahey. *How the Way We Talk Can Change the Way We Work: Seven Languages for Transformation.* San Francisco: Jossey-Bass, 2001.

Kenyon, Tom, M.A. *Brain States.* Lithia Springs, GA: New Leaf, 2001.

Kirsch, Daniel L., and Marshall Gilula. "Cranial Electrotherapy Stimulation in the Treatment of Depression—Part 1: Practical Pain Management," 7, no. 4 (2007): 33–41. Part 2: 7, no. 5 (2007): 32–40.

Larson, Joan Mathews, Ph.D. *Depression-Free, Naturally.* New York: Ballantine, 1999.

————. *Seven Weeks to Sobriety.* New York: Ballantine, 1997.

Leonard, George. *Mastery: The Keys to Success and Long-Term Fulfillment.* New York: Penguin Books, 1992.

————, and Michael Murphy. *The Life We Are Given: A Long-term Program for Realizing the Potential of Body, Mind, Heart, and Soul.* New York: Tarcher/Putnam, 1995.

Lesser, Michael, M.D. *The Brain Chemistry Diet.* New York: Putnam's Sons, 2002.

Levine, Noah. *Dharma Punx: A Memoir.* New York: HarperCollins, 2003.

Lynch, David. *Catching the Big Fish: Meditation, Consciousness, and Creativity.* New York: Penguin, 2006.

Manchester, William. *The Last Lion: Winston Spencer Churchill, Visions of Glory, 1874–1932.* New York: Little, Brown, 1983.

————. *The Last Lion: Winston Spencer Churchill, Alone, 1932–1940.* New York: Dell, 1988.

Maslow, Abraham. *Toward a Psychology of Being.* New York: Wiley and Sons, 1968, 1999.

May, Gerald, M.D. *Addiction and Grace: Love and Spirituality in the Healing of Addictions.* New York: HarperCollins, 1988.

McCauley, Kevin T. *Addiction: New Understanding, Fresh Hope, Real Healing.* Audio CD. Salt Lake City: The Institute for Addiction Study, 2007.

————. *The Disease Model of Addiction—Part 1.* Audio CD. Salt Lake City: The Institute for Addiction Study, 2007.

————. *The Disease Model of Addiction—Part 2*. Audio CD. Salt Lake City: The Institute for Addiction Study, 2007.

————. *Pleasure Unwoven: An Explanation of the Brain Disease of Addiction*. DVD. Directed by K. McCauley, produced by Jim Clegg of the Institute for Addiction Study, 2010.

Miller, Melvin E., and Susanne Cook-Greuter, eds. *Creativity, Spirituality, and Transcendence: Paths to Integrity and Wisdom in the Mature Self*. Stamford, CT: Ablex, 2000.

————. *Transcendence and Mature Thought in Adulthood: The Further Reaches of Adult Development*. Lanham, MD: Rowman and Littlefield, 1994.

Miller, William R., and Janet C'de Baca. *Quantum Change: When Epiphanies and Sudden Insights Transform Ordinary Lives*. New York: Guilford, 2001.

Miller, William R., and Stephen Rollnick. *Motivational Interviewing*. New York: Guilford, 2002.

Murphy, Michael. *The Future of the Body: Explorations into the Further Evolution of Human Nature*. New York: Tarcher/Perigee, 1993.

The National Center on Addiction and Substance Abuse at Columbia University. *Women under the Influence*. Johns Hopkins University Press, 2006.

The National Center on Addiction and Substance Abuse at Columbia University (CASA) Press Releases: 2010. "Behind Bars II: Substance Abuse and America's Prison Population." Duran, Lauren and Sulaiman Beg, contacts. CASAColumbia.org: News Room: Press Releases.

Newport, John, Ph.D. *The Wellness-Recovery Connection*. Deerfield Beach: Health Communications, 2004.

Olds, J. and P. Milner. "Positive Reinforcement Produced by Electrical Stimulation of Septal Area and Other Regions of Rat Brain." *Journal of Comparative and Physiological Psychology* 47 (1956): 419–427.

————. "Pleasure Centers in the Brain." *Scientific American* (October 1956). Reprinted in S. Coopersmith, ed., *Frontiers of Psychological Research* (pp. 54–59). San Francisco: Freeman, 1966.

Oster, G. (1973). "Auditory Beats in the Brain." *Scientific American* 229, no. 4 (1973): 94–102.

Palmer, Helen. *The Enneagram: Understanding Yourself and the Others in Your Life*. New York: HarperCollins, 1991.

————. *The Enneagram in Love and Work: Understanding Your Intimate and Business Relationships*. New York: HarperCollins, 1993.

Peniston, E. G., and P. J. Kulkowski. "Alpha-Theta Brainwave Training and Beta-endorphin Levels in Alcoholics." *Alcoholism* 13 (1989): 271–79.

Phillips, Bill, *Body for Life*. New York: HarperCollins, 1999.

Phillips, Shawn, *Strength for Life*. New York: Ballantine Books, 2008.

Prentiss, Chris. *The Alcoholism Addiction Cure: A Holistic Approach to Total Recovery*. California: Power, 2005.

Prigogine, Ilya, and Isabelle Stengers. *Order out of Chaos: Man's New Dialogue with Nature*. New York: Bantam, 1984.

Riso, Don Richard, and Russ Hudson. *Personality Types: Using the Enneagram for Self-Discovery*. New York: Houghton Mifflin, 1996.

————. *The Wisdom of the Enneagram: The Complete Guide to Psychological and Spiritual Growth for the Nine Personality Types*. New York: Bantam, 1999.

Rohr, Richard. *Everything Belongs: The Gift of Contemplative Prayer*. New York: Crossroad, 1999, 2003.

Russell, K. C. (2007). "The Therapeutic Alliance." Summary of research in the Outdoor Behavioral Healthcare Research Cooperative from 1999–2006. Technical Report 2, February 2007, Outdoor Behavioral Healthcare Research Cooperative, College of Education and Human Development, University of Minnesota, Minneapolis, MN. 52 pp.

Schlitz, Marilyn Mandala, Cassandra Vieten, and Tina Amorok. *Living Deeply: The Art and Science of Transformation in Everyday Life*. Oakland: New Harbinger Publications and Noetic Books, 2007.

Schwartz, Jeffrey M., M.D. and Sharon Begley. *The Mind and the Brain: Neuroplasticity and the Power of Mental Force*. New York: HarperCollins, 2002.

Sears, Barry, Ph.D. *Enter the Zone*. New York: HarperCollins, 1995.

————. *Mastering the Zone*. New York: HarperCollins, 1997.

Selye, Hans. *The Stress of Life*. McGraw-Hill, 2nd edition, 1978.

————. *Stress of My Life: A Scientist's Memoirs*. Van Nostrand Reinhold, 1979.

————. *Stress without Distress*. Lippincott Williams & Wilkins, 1st edition, 1974.

Shenk, David. *The Genius in All of Us: New Insights into Genetics, Talent, and IQ*. New York: Random House, 2009.

Siegel, Daniel J., M.D. *Mindsight: The New Science of Transformation*. New York: Random House, 2010.

Slaga, Thomas J., and Robin Keuneke. *The Detox Revolution*. New York: McGraw Hill Books, 2003.

Smith, Paul R. *Integral Christianity: The Spirit's Call to Evolve*. St. Paul, MN: Paragon House, 2011.

Smith, Ray B., Ph.D. *Cranial Electrotherapy Stimulation: Its First Fifty Years, Plus Three: A Monograph*. Mustang, Oklahoma: Tate, 2007.

Sommers, Christina Hoff. *The War against Boys*. New York: Simon and Schuster, 2000.

Sturza, Marisa L., and Rebecca Campbell. "An Exploratory Study of Rape Survivors' Prescription Drug Use as a Means of Coping with Sexual Assault." *Psychology of Women Quarterly* 21, no. 4 (Dec. 1, 2005): 353–363.

Swimme, Brian Thomas. *The Universe Is a Green Dragon: A Cosmic Creation Story*. Rochester, VT: Bear, 1984.

Tarnas, Richard. *The Passion of the Western Mind: Understanding the Ideas That Have Shaped Our World View*. New York: Ballantine Books, 1991.

Volpicelli, Joseph, and Maia Szalavitz. *Recovery Options: The Complete Guide: How You and Your Loved Ones Can Understand and Treat Alcohol and Other Drug Problems*. New York: John Wiley & Sons, 2000.

Wahbeh, H., Calabrese, C., Zwickey, H. "Binaural Beat Technology in Humans: A Pilot Study to Assess Psychological and Physiologic Effects." *Journal of Alternative and Complementary Medicine* 13, no. 1 (2007): 25–32.

Wahbeh, H., C. Calabrese, H. Zwickey, and J. Zajdel. "Binaural Beat Technology in Humans: A Pilot Study to Assess Neuropsychologic, Physiologic, and Electroencephalographic Effects." *Journal of Alternative and Complementary Medicine* 13, no. 2 (2007): 199–206.

Walsh, Roger N., M.D. *Essential Spirituality: The 7 Central Practices to Awaken Heart and Mind*. New York: Wiley and Sons, 1999.

Weil, Andrew, M.D. *Eating Well for Optimum Health*. New York: Knopf, 2000.

Wilber, Ken. *The Atman Project: A Transpersonal View of Human Development*. Quest Books, 2nd Edition, 1996.

———. *Boomeritis: A Novel That Will Set You Free*. Boston: Shambhala, 2002.

———. *A Brief History of Everything*. Boston: Shambhala, 1996, 2000.

———. *The Eye of Spirit: An Integral Vision for a World Gone Slightly Mad*. Boston: Shambhala, 2001, 2000.

———. Foreword to *Integral Medicine: A Noetic Reader*, at http://www.kenwilber.com/writings/index?category=Forewords.

———. *Grace and Grit: Spirituality and Healing in the Life and Death of Treya Killam Wilber*. Boston: Shambhala, 1991, 2000.

———. *The Integral Operating System: Version 1.0*. CDs, DVD, workbook. Boulder: Sounds True, 2005.

———. *Integral Psychology: Consciousness, Spirit, Psychology, Therapy*. Boston: Shambhala, 2000.

———. *Integral Spirituality: A Startling New Role for Religion in the Modern and Post-modern World*. Integral Books, an imprint of Shambhala Publications, 2006.

———. *The Integral Vision: A Very Short Introduction to the Revolutionary Integral Approach to Life, God, the Universe, and Everything*. Boston: Shambhala, 2007.

———. "Introduction to Integral Theory and Practice: The AQAL Map," published on the integralnaked.org website.

———. *The Marriage of Sense and Soul: Integrating Science and Religion*. New York: Random House, 1998.

———. *One Taste: Daily Reflections on Integral Spirituality*. Boston: Shambhala, 2000.

———. *The One Two Three of God*. Audio CD. Boulder: Sounds True, 2006.

———. *Sex, Ecology, Spirituality: The Spirit of Evolution*. Boston: Shambhala, 1995, 2000.

———, Terry Patton, Adam Leonard, and Marco Morelli. *Integral Life Practice: A Twenty-first-Century Blueprint for Physical Health, Emotional Balance, Mental Clarity, and Spiritual Awakening*. Boston: Integral Books, an imprint of Shambhala Publications, 2008.

Index